Human Vaccines

Emerging Technologies in Design and Development

T0318734

Edited by

Kayvon Modjarrad, MD, PhD

Associate Director, Emerging Infectious Disease Threats,
Military HIV Research Program/Walter Reed Army Institute of Research,
Bethesda, MD, USA

Wayne C. Koff, PhD

President and CEO,
Human Vaccines Project, New York, NY, USA

ELSEVIER

AMSTERDAM • BOSTON • HEIDELBERG • LONDON
NEW YORK • OXFORD • PARIS • SAN DIEGO
SAN FRANCISCO • SINGAPORE • SYDNEY • TOKYO
Academic Press is an imprint of Elsevier

Academic Press is an imprint of Elsevier
125 London Wall, London EC2Y 5AS, United Kingdom
525 B Street, Suite 1800, San Diego, CA 92101-4495, United States
50 Hampshire Street, 5th Floor, Cambridge, MA 02139, United States
The Boulevard, Langford Lane, Kidlington, Oxford OX5 1GB, United Kingdom

British Library Cataloguing-in-Publication Data
A catalogue record for this book is available from the British Library

Library of Congress Cataloging-in-Publication Data
A catalog record for this book is available from the Library of Congress

ISBN: 978-0-12-802302-0

For Information on all Academic Press publications
visit our website at https://www.elsevier.com

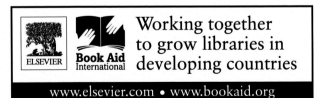

Working together
to grow libraries in
developing countries

www.elsevier.com • www.bookaid.org

Publisher: Sara Tenney
Acquisition Editor: Linda Versteeg-Buschman
Editorial Project Manager: Halima Williams
Production Project Manager: Karen East and Kirsty Halterman
Designer: Victoria Pearson

Typeset by MPS Limited, Chennai, India

Human Vaccines

Contents

Part III
Immune Monitoring

List of Contributors

C.B. Buck Center for Cancer Research, NCI, National Institutes of Health, Bethesda, MD, United States

C.B. Creech Vanderbilt University, Nashville, TN, United States

E. Del Tordello GSK Vaccines, Siena, Italy

I. Delany GSK Vaccines, Siena, Italy

K.M. Edwards Vanderbilt University, Nashville, TN, United States

M.A. Eller US Military HIV Research Program, Walter Reed Army Institute of Research, Silver Spring, MD, United States; The Henry M. Jackson Foundation for the Advancement of Military Medicine, Inc., Bethesda, MD, United States

S. Gaudieri Murdoch University, Murdoch, WA, Australia; University of Western Australia, Crawley, WA, Australia; Vanderbilt University, Nashville, TN, United States

P.B. Gilbert Fred Hutchinson Cancer Research Center, Seattle, WA, United States; University of Washington, Seattle, WA, United States

R. Gottardo Fred Hutchinson Cancer Research Center, Seattle, WA, United States; University of Washington, Seattle, WA, United States

M. John Murdoch University, Murdoch, WA, Australia; University of Western Australia, Crawley, WA, Australia

M. Kanekiyo Vaccine Research Center, NIAID, National Institutes of Health, Bethesda, MD, United States

S. Mallal Murdoch University, Murdoch, WA, Australia; Vanderbilt University, Nashville, TN, United States

T.A. Moody Duke University, Durham, NC, United States

L. Morris National Institute for Communicable Diseases, Johannesburg, South Africa

C.L. Parks The International AIDS Vaccine Initiative, Brooklyn, NY, United States

R. Rappuoli GSK Vaccines, Siena, Italy

M. Rolland US Military HIV Research Program, Walter Reed Army Institute of Research, Silver Spring, MD, United States; The Henry M. Jackson Foundation for the Advancement of Military Medicine, Inc., Bethesda, MD, United States

Foreword

It is a clichéd but undeniable claim that vaccines have been one of the most effective medical interventions in human history. However, the science of vaccine development has evolved considerably over the years since Pasteur created the first vaccines in his laboratory. Attenuation or inactivation of whole bacteria and viruses by physicochemical means served vaccine development well for the earliest products.[1,2] Gradually, over the course of the 20th century, an evolution in attenuation techniques took place. Pathogens were passaged in cell culture or in animals, allowing for the selection of less virulent strains. Chemical inactivation also became more precise, improving the immunogenicity of toxoids or whole organisms. Later, a common strategy was formulated to develop vaccines based on proteins or polysaccharides that elicited protective immune responses during natural infection. The advent of genetic engineering made it possible to produce large quantities of those protective antigens. These basic techniques worked well in situations where relatively straightforward antibody or cellular responses to single antigens were protective or where replicating attenuated organisms could induce protection without disease.

As we move further into the 21st century it has become clear that a deeper understanding of antigenic structure and immune responses is necessary for future success. Each pathogen presents a unique set of challenges for vaccine development, but there are common deficiencies in defining and developing immunity against all infectious diseases that can be addressed by emerging technologies. The inability, thus far, to produce highly efficacious vaccines against HIV or tuberculosis is emblematic of these deficiencies, but vaccine development against other diseases is also impeded by our collective ignorance. A prime example is that of respiratory syncytial virus (RSV), the first and second most important causes of respiratory disease in infants and the elderly, respectively.[3–6] Although an effective vaccine against RSV should produce functional antibodies, the epitopes that are important for neutralization are not present on all forms of the virus's surface fusion protein.[7] A cellular response may also be important to protection, particularly in the elderly, but we do not know whether CD4+ or CD8+ T cells are more important or if they might actually be immunopathogenic rather than immunoprotective. In addition, we do not know why natural reinfection with RSV is so frequent. To put it another way, what is the defect in natural immunity to RSV?

Another striking example of our ignorance of immune correlates of protection relates to pertussis vaccines. Neither whole cell nor acellular vaccines give long-lasting immunity, although the latter clearly gives less durable protection.[8,9] How can we generate the kind of T helper cell responses that will boost and prolong B and T cell effector memory in the case of infections with a short incubation period and central memory in setting of infections with a long incubation period. The value of effector CD8+ T cells is also becoming more apparent across various vaccines, including those against HIV.[10] When it comes to antibody responses, great strides have been made in their characterization, but there remains a great need for more detailed understanding of antibody functions. Our artificial in vitro neutralization tests do not reflect all functions of protective antibodies. For example, we know that antibody avidity and isotype influence immunity[11,12] and that non-neutralizing antibodies acting through antibody dependent cellular cytoxicity are also important to protection from disease; but none of these mechanisms are captured on our standard immunoassays.

As vaccine-elicited immunity is better elucidated, improved platforms for vaccine delivery are also going forward in parallel. Vectors, one of the more versatile vaccine platforms, are defined as microbes or nucleic acids carrying information for a pathogen protein that induces a protective response. The simplest case is a DNA plasmid coding for a surface protein such as HIV gp120.[13] More recently, RNA segments have also come into play, expressing proteins, for example, that are important for protection against cytomegalovirus.[14] Viral (e.g., adenoviruses, poxviruses) and bacterial (e.g., BCG) vectors are the most widely used, expressing specific proteins during either complete replication or a single cycle of defective replication. This strategy has been used most extensively for HIV vaccines.[15,16] The biggest challenge with vectors is the induction of immunity to the vector itself, precluding the use of multiple doses in one vaccination regimen. The way around this impediment has been through the use of regimens of heterologous vectors, the so-called prime-boost strategy. Typically, two doses of a DNA- or adenovirus-based vector are administered, followed by a poxvirus vector or the protein of interest. Even if we overcome the problem of vector immunity, we still do not understand why prime-boost regimens work so well. Confounding the issue even more is that all vectors are equally immunogenic. Adenovirus vectors tend to generate higher CD8+ T cell responses, whereas poxvirus vectors are better at generating CD4+ T cell responses.[17,18] Cytomegalovirus vectors induce CD8+ responses that vary with the genetic content of the insert.[10] This is where systems biology and basic immunology could give us crucial information to enable better understanding and use of vectors.

Among the many emerging technologies, the use of genomics, sometimes called reverse vaccinology, has great potential in offering up new antigenic targets for vaccine development. This technology has already yielded one vaccine, meningococcus Group B,[19] but there are many other bacteria and some large viruses that could undergo genomic analysis for the purpose of identifying immunogenic epitopes. In fact, organisms with large genomes are likely to have both "genes" that induce protective immune responses and "genes" that inhibit the host from generating protective immune responses. Genomics should thus permit selection of the right mixture of antigens. Vaccines against staphylococcus, as an example, could greatly benefit from reverse vaccinology. Virus like particle (VLP) technologies have also emerged in recent decades as a powerful tool for vaccine development. The VLP human papillomavirus vaccines are among the most safe and efficacious vaccines available, paving the way for the same strategy to be applied to other viruses whose correlate of protection is associated with a single surface protein. Norovirus VLP vaccines appear to be working well; however, the organism may mutate sufficiently to require periodic updates of vaccine antigens.[20] One solution to pathogen mutability could be the use of VLPs that present an array of heterologous antigens.[21] Nanoparticle vaccines may be an attractive alternative to VLPs as they can also present multiple antigens, but enter cells more easily, including those in the intestinal tract, thus facilitating more robust mucosal immune responses.[22–24]

Notable among all the technological developments in vaccinology is the growing tendency to move away from live attenuated vaccines, largely owing to theoretical or actual safety concerns. The consequence of this trend is the need for more powerful adjuvants to nonreplicating antigens. This is an area rich in possibilities—already progressing through the use of toll-like receptor (TLR) agonists—but one that will require careful consideration of safety in general but also with specificity to the genetics of the vaccinated population, a concept that has been termed "adversomics."[25] Thus, adjuvants may have to be chosen with regard to the immunogenetic group of the vaccinee.

All of this requires that we learn much more about how to induce adaptive immune responses that are not only protective but durable. We have much to learn about the breadth and memory of B and T cell responses before we can mimic the solid protection that often follows natural infection. Indeed, in some cases like RSV and malaria, we wish to do better than natural immunity. A major collaborative Human Vaccines Project is needed to reach these goals.[26] Predicting the course of vaccinology is probably no more certain than predicting the weather. Be that as it may, I foresee that no future vaccine will be developed without a profound understanding of the structure of the antigens used. The most successful vaccine antigens will contain only those portions that generate protective responses, although vaccines to inhibit certain adverse effects such as allergic responses could also be possible if we identify the right epitopes.[27] In the coming decades, vaccines that induce durable, protective immunity will also be based on knowledge of how best to stimulate T follicular helper cells, plasmablasts, and where required, CD8 + effector T cell responses. Innate immunity elicited by vaccination will also need be better characterized, as it will not only influence protection but have nonspecific effects on other pathogens as well.[28] All vaccines likely will need to be adjuvanted to stimulate both innate and adaptive immune responses.

There is a long and growing list of diseases for which vaccines are needed. Ultimately, the advent of new strategies and technologies to induce robust immunity bodes well for the future of vaccine research and development. However, beyond the need for advances in basic science, we must learn better ways to demonstrate safety and efficacy of vaccines with greater cost- and time-efficiency. So the vaccine enterprise has much to do in order to reap the fruits of new discoveries. This volume speaks to how we can build into on vaccinology's solid foundation of the past hundred years and recapitulate our successes in the coming century.

S.A. Plotkin MD
University of Pennsylvania, Philadelphia, PA, United States

REFERENCES

1. Plotkin S. History of vaccination. *Proc Natl Acad Sci USA* 2014;**111**(34):12283−7.
2. Plotkin SA, Plotkin SL. The development of vaccines: how the past led to the future. *Nat Rev Microbiol* 2011;**9**(12):889−93.
3. Karron RA, Buchholz UM, Collins PL. Live-attenuated respiratory syncytial virus vaccine. *Curr Top Microbiol immunol* 2015;**372**:259−84.
4. Hall CB, Weinberg GA, Iwane MK, et al. The burden of respiratory syncytial virus infection in young children. *N Engl J Med* 2009;**360**(6):588−98.
5. Falsey AR, Walsh EE. Respiratory syncytial virus infection in adults. *Clin Microbiol Rev* 2000;**13**(3):371−84.
6. Espinoza JA, Bueno SM, Riedel CA, Kalergis AM. Induction of protective effector immunity to prevent pathogenesis caused by the respiratory syncytial virus. Implications on therapy and vaccine design. *Immunology* 2014;**143**(1):1−12.
7. McLellan JS, Chen M, Joyce MG, et al. Structure-based design of a fusion glycoprotein vaccine for respiratory syncytial virus. *Science* 2013;**342**(6158):592−8.
8. Meade BD, Plotkin SA, Locht C. Possible options for new pertussis vaccines. *J Infect Dis* 2014;**209**(Suppl 1):S24−7.
9. McGirr A, Fisman DN. Duration of pertussis immunity after DTaP immunization: a meta-analysis. *Pediatrics* 2015;**135**(Jan):1729.
10. Hansen SG, Sacha JB, Hughes CM, et al. Cytomegalovirus vectors violate CD8 + T cell epitope recognition paradigms. *Science* 2013;**340**(6135):1237874.
11. Yates NL, Liao HX, Fong Y, et al. Vaccine-induced Env V1-V2 IgG3 correlates with lower HIV-1 infection risk and declines soon after vaccination. *Sci Transl Med* 2014;**6** (228). 228ra239.
12. Excler JL, Ake J, Robb ML, Kim JH, Plotkin SA. Nonneutralizing functional antibodies: a new "old" paradigm for HIV vaccines. *Clin Vaccine Immunol* 2014;**21**(8):1023−36.

13. Ugen K, Weiner DB. DNA vaccines onward and upward! 20 years and counting! Highlights of the DNA vaccines 2012 meeting. *Hum Vaccin Immunother* 2013;**9** (10):2038−40.

14. Brito LA, Kommareddy S, Maione D, et al. Self-amplifying mRNA vaccines. *Adv Genet* 2015;**89**:179−233.

15. de Cassan SC, Draper SJ. Recent advances in antibody-inducing poxviral and adenoviral vectored vaccine delivery platforms for difficult disease targets. *Expert Rev Vaccines* 2013;**12**(4):365−78.

16. Majhen D, Calderon H, Chandra N, et al. Adenovirus-based vaccines for fighting infectious diseases and cancer: progress in the field. *Hum Gene Ther* 2014;**25**(4):301−17.

17. Thiele F, Tao S, Zhang Y, et al. MVA-infected dendritic cells present CD4 + T-cell epitopes by endogenous MHC class II presentation pathways. *J Virol* 2014;**89**(5). 03244-14.

18. Johnson JA, Barouch DH, Baden LR. Nonreplicating vectors in HIV vaccines. *Curr Opin HIV AIDS* 2013;**8**(5):412−20.

19. Seib KL, Zhao X, Rappuoli R. Developing vaccines in the era of genomics: a decade of reverse vaccinology. *Clin Microbiol Infect* 2012;**18**(Suppl 5):109−16.

20. Ramani S, Atmar RL, Estes MK. Epidemiology of human noroviruses and updates on vaccine development. *Curr Opin Gastroenterol* 2014;**30**(1):25−33.

21. Cuburu N, Wang K, Goodman KN, et al. Topical herpes simplex virus 2 (HSV-2) vaccination with human papillomavirus vectors expressing gB/gD ectodomains induces genital-tissue-resident memory CD8+ T cells and reduces genital disease and viral shedding after HSV-2 challenge. *J Virol* 2015;**89**(1):83−96.

22. Zhao L, Seth A, Wibowo N, et al. Nanoparticle vaccines. *Vaccine* 2014;**32**(3):327−37.

23. Sharma R, Agrawal U, Mody N, Vyas SP. Polymer nanotechnology based approaches in mucosal vaccine delivery: challenges and opportunities. *Biotechnol Adv* 2014;**33**(1):64−79.

24. Marasini N, Skwarczynski M, Toth I. Oral delivery of nanoparticle-based vaccines. *Expert Rev Vaccines* 2014;**13**(11):1361−76.

25. Poland GA, Kennedy RB, McKinney BA, et al. Vaccinomics, adversomics, and the immune response network theory: individualized vaccinology in the 21st century. *Semin Immunol* 2013;**25**(2):89−103.

26. Koff WC, Gust ID, Plotkin SA. Toward a human vaccines project. *Nat Immunol* 2014;**15** (7):589−92.

27. Moise L, Terry F, Gutierrez AH, et al. Smarter vaccine design will circumvent regulatory T cell-mediated evasion in chronic HIV and HCV infection. *Front Microbiol* 2014;**5**:502.

28. Aaby P, Kollmann TR, Benn CS. Nonspecific effects of neonatal and infant vaccination: public-health, immunological and conceptual challenges. *Nat Immunol* 2014;**15**(10):895−9.

Part I

Designing Vaccines From a New Starting Point

Chapter 1

Broadly Neutralizing Antibodies

L. Morris[1] and T.A. Moody[2]

[1]*National Institute for Communicable Diseases, Johannesburg, South Africa,*
[2]*Duke University, Durham, NC, United States*

The antibody response to human pathogens is generally robust, highly specific, long-lasting and, in many cases, able to clear infection. The initial encounter between a naïve B cell receptor (BCR) and a foreign antigen activates B cell clonal lineages that subsequently undergo somatic hypermutation and selection in a process that increases antibody affinity. In most cases, the first detectable antibody response in the plasma is of the IgM class, switching to IgG and IgA classes within several weeks after infection. As most high-affinity antibodies develop, B cells engage CD4$^+$ T follicular helper cells in germinal centers and exit as plasmablasts. Intermediate IgM and class-switched memory B cells are also released into circulation at predictable intervals during the process.[1,2] Large quantities of antibodies are produced by short-lived plasmablasts that are found in the circulation during an acute infection. These cells appear in particularly high numbers in response to human immunodeficiency virus type 1 (HIV-1), although the vast majority are not HIV-1-specific because of extensive B cell hyperactivation that is a hallmark of the disease.[3] For those infections that are cleared, resolution is associated with a decline in the circulating plasmablast and retention memory B cell pools that are available for recall upon subsequent exposures. Consequently, secondary responses are more rapid, generate higher affinity antibodies and mediate protection against reinfection or at least severe disease.

The BCR is an integral membrane form of the antibody that is specific to each B cell. Antibodies are heterodimeric proteins consisting of heavy and light chains that combine to form a basic "Y" shaped structure. Both surface-bound and secreted antibodies have a compartmentalized construction that includes a region able to recognize antigens. The process of antibody gene rearrangement[4] results in a large array of antibody binding sites that are further diversified by somatic hypermutation.[5] Each antibody

Human Vaccines: Emerging Technologies in Design and Development.
DOI: http://dx.doi.org/10.1016/B978-0-12-802302-0.00012-1
3

contains two antigen recognition sites making up each arm of the "Y" shaped structure. These portions—the "fragment antigen binding" or Fab regions—are the primary focus of efforts to isolate and characterize human antibodies. The third major functional and structural component of an antibody is the "fragment constant" or Fc region that defines antibody isotypes and subclasses. It interacts with effector arms of the immune system either by binding receptor molecules (e.g., plasma complement proteins) or by binding cell surface receptors on effector cells (e.g., NK cells). These Fc-mediated effector functions likely play an important role in a number of infections as they enhance the antiviral efficacy of antibodies. Antibody functions can be further manipulated through recombinant engineering of the Fc region, either by mutating amino acid residues, changing glycosylation patterns, or both. This has been a common practice for the development of monoclonal antibodies (mAbs) in clinical use.

The most important antiviral function of an antibody is pathogen neutralization, mediated through the specificity afforded by the Fab portion. Neutralization is a measure of the ability of an antibody to prevent pathogen entry into a cell, and it is thought to occur by a variety of mechanisms that include steric hindrance, target dissociation and promotion of structural inflexibility in the pathogen's surface proteins. Effective neutralization is dependent on antibodies that target functionally active sites. Those antibodies that recognize highly conserved regions in the pathogen proteins are more likely to be broadly neutralizing and, therefore, most desirable to elicit when designing a vaccine.

The isolation of broadly neutralizing antibodies has been a major focus of efforts to develop vaccines against many pathogens, including HIV, influenza, respiratory syncytial virus (RSV).[6] In addition to their roles in preventing, reducing and clearing infection, neutralizing antibodies serve as a correlate of protection for most human vaccines.[7] Thus, studying the targets of protective antibodies could result in improvements to existing vaccines or the development of novel ones. Furthermore, isolation, detailed biochemical characterization, epitope mapping and structural modeling of mAbs could pave the way for the development of vaccines and therapeutics for a range of diseases for which no interventions are currently available.

IDENTIFICATION OF BROADLY CROSS-REACTIVE ANTIBODIES IN HUMAN DONORS

The detection of serum antibody responses to a pathogen of interest is generally a good indication of the presence of circulating antigen-specific memory B cells and/or plasmablasts from which the mAbs are isolated. In the case of HIV 1, suitable donors have been identified by screening large volumes of sera for their ability to neutralize viral isolates of multiple subtypes.[8−12] This process has resulted in the isolation of a large number of highly potent, broadly neutralizing antibodies to HIV-1.[13,14] A similar approach has been applied to the isolation of a mAb that cross-reacts with RSV and metapneumovirus. In this example healthy donors with presumed past infection, by one or both of these viruses, were screened for serum activity against both viruses.[15] Broadly neutralizing influenza mAbs have also been isolated and have largely come from studies of pandemic survivors,[16–18] experimental and licensed vaccine recipients[19–21] and experimentally infected volunteers.[20] Since antigen-specific antibodies persist in the circulation for many years,[22] donor screenings can be performed long after infection, as was the case among 1918 Spanish influenza pandemic survivors.[18]

The characterization of antibody specificities responsible for serum neutralizing activity greatly facilitates efforts to isolate mAbs of interest. However, mapping antibody specificity is confounded by the fact that neutralizing antibodies are a minor component of the polyclonal antibody response. Nevertheless, multiple techniques have been developed for this purpose and used successfully. Peptide arrays, for example, screen antibody specificities through the presentation of overlapping peptides. Although they have been used for a number of infections, the general approach is limited by the fact that most broadly neutralizing antibodies recognize conformational epitopes and glycans that are not represented in the arrays.[23] The use of epitope-ablating mutants has also been helpful in mapping neutralizing antibody specificities, particularly those that target glycans on the HIV-1 envelope glycoprotein.[24–26] Depletion of plasma neutralizing activity through protein or peptide adsorption provides additional information for the design of soluble antigens that can bait antibodies of interest.[27,28]

The availability of large neutralization datasets has aided in the design of bioinformatic algorithms to predict specificities of serum samples, particularly in the case of HIV-1.[29–31] However, both experimental and computational epitope mapping methods are hampered by the presence of antibodies against multiple or undefined targets; in these cases mAb isolation may be necessary. While many of these technologies have been developed for the study of HIV-1, they have not been limited to this pathogen but applied others, like dengue virus, with great success.[32]

ISOLATION OF MONOCLONAL ANTIBODIES USING B CELL CULTURE TECHNOLOGIES

The first generalizable technique for isolating monoclonal antibodies was reported in 1975 by Kohler and Milstein.[33] This Nobel-prize winning pair fused an immortalized myeloma cell line (P3-X63Ag8) with mouse splenocytes to generate so-called hybridomas: stable cell-lines that secrete antibodies in culture. This process has led to the development of many mAbs that are still in use as immunologic reagents. Although the method represented a significant technological advance at the time, it carries a number of limitations.

Hybridoma technology depends on a high frequency of B cells that make the antibodies of interest. It has a generally low efficiency of hybridization between immortalized myeloma cells and splenocytes, and extension of the process from murine to human B cells has not been very successful.

Many large-quantity human mAb production protocols have been based on the transformation of B cells with Epstein-Barr virus (EBV), a human herpes virus with B cell tropism.[34] However, EBV entry into B cells is partially dependent upon CD21 expression,[35] which appears to be linked to in vitro B cell survival and proliferation. Over the past 20 years, investigations into B cell activation have found potent activators such as CD40L, IL-21, and CpG improve transformation efficiency either on their own or in concert with EBV. After activation, purified memory B cells can then be cultured over a short period (10−14 days), at which time supernatant is collected and screened for pathogen (usually virus) neutralization. High-throughput functional screening methods now make it easier to scan a large numbers of cultures in order to detect rare B cell populations[36,37] (Fig. 1.1A). As this technique is predicated on detecting functional antibody activity, donors must be selected carefully for their capacity to neutralize viruses at low antibody concentrations. Some of the most potent HIV-1 mAbs ever isolated have been found through this process, likely because of the stringency of the functional screening step.[37−39] A major advantage of using B cell culture to isolate mAbs is that the target epitope does not need to be predefined, thus enabling the isolation of antibodies that recognize new, previously unrecognized targets. Still, culturing memory B cells is relatively labor-intensive, requires large amounts of space and laboratory equipment, is prone to technical complications such as cell overgrowth and death and may result in antibody class switching during the culture period.[40] Multiple antibody lineages in one donor target the glycan-V3 supersite of the HIV-1 envelope glycoprotein and display a preference for quaternary binding.[40a]

ISOLATION OF mABs BY ANTIGEN-SPECIFIC SORTING

The identification of target epitopes by mapping antibody specificity allows for the design of highly specific antigens to sort out single B cells (Fig. 1.1B). One of the earliest and most successful applications of this technology involved the use of the resurfaced core 3 (RSC3) antigen of the HIV-1 envelope to isolate VRC01, a broad and potent CD4 binding site (CD4bs) antibody.[41] Interestingly, the majority of mAbs that were isolated by these means use a restricted set of germline genes.[42]

A number of techniques for sorting antigen-specific B cells have since been developed, but all of them display antigens that must be bound by immunoglobulins fixed to the B cell surface. As each method has particular advantages and disadvantages (Table 1.1), selection of the most suitable method depends greatly on the antigenic target. The simplest approach uses linear synthetic peptides that have a sequence motif (e.g.,

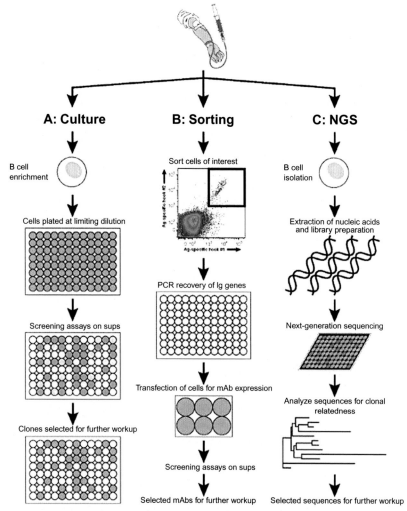

FIGURE 1.1 Schematic of the methods used to isolate monoclonal antibodies: (A) B cell culture, (B) B cell sorting, and (C) Paired reads of the immunoglobulin repertoire.

biotin) that can be designed in a manner that permits detection by a flow cytometer (e.g., fluorochrome-derivatized streptavidin). This technique was first used to identify a class of autoantibodies recognizing a mimetope of double stranded DNA[43] and subsequently used to isolate an antibody directed against the membrane proximal external region (MPER) of the HIV-1 envelope glycoprotein, gp41.[44] Peptide-based MPER reagents have also been used to characterize immune tolerance in mouse models,[45,46] work that has ultimately led to the identification of the autoantigen responsible for the

TABLE 1.1 Techniques for Isolation of Antigen-Specific B Cells

Technique	Advantages	Disadvantages
Linear peptides	• Simplicity • Ease of manufacture	• Depends on antibody recognition of linear sequence • Cannot be used for discontinuous or quaternary epitopes
Monomeric proteins	• Expression of epitopes in a more native conformation	• Requires protein synthesis • Cannot be used for quaternary epitopes
Multimeric proteins (e.g., trimers)	• Expression of epitopes in a more native conformation	• Requires the production of stable multimeric complexes
Virus-like particles	• Epitopes presented in situ on the surface of the particle, presumably in a native conformation	• Particle production can be difficult • Epitopes can be expressed in nonnative conformations • Can select for B cells reactive against other antigens on the particle
Cell-expressed antigens	• Epitopes presented in situ on the surface of the cell, presumably in a native conformation	• Requires production of cells expressing the antigen, can select for B cells reactive with other antigens on the cell • Relatively low specificity for isolated mAbs
Culture-based B cell recovery	• No need for prior knowledge of epitope targets • Screening can be based on functional assays (e.g., neutralization)	• Labor and resource intensive • Loss of cells of interest possible through contamination or outgrowth of irrelevant cells

regulation of this antibody class.[47] Although this technique is highly specific for epitopes presented as a linear peptide sequence, it comes at some cost. First, the method does not allow for the presentation of discontinuous or structurally complex epitopes. Second, it is poorly suited for in-depth characterization of antibodies generated in response to vaccination or infection.

Recombinant proteins are increasingly being used as baits to isolate antigen-specific B cells. For example, the highly specific CD4bs antibodies were isolated through a differential sort where the second screening antigen lacked the epitope of interest (e.g., RSC3 proteins with mutations at position

368 or 371 ablated the CD4 binding site).[41] A similar approach used a chimeric protein to isolate a strain-specific neutralizing antibody against the α2 helix of HIV-1 gp120.[48] Proteins derived from vaccine trial immunogens have also been used to isolate cells from vaccine recipients.[49,50] While these isolated mAbs are not broadly neutralizing, they have been helpful in resolving potential mechanisms of protection.[51] Unlike linear peptides, whole proteins display discontinuous or conformational epitopes that increase the likelihood of isolating B cells that recognize complex targets. Epitopes that are present at the interface of protein subunits are particularly useful for B cell isolation when configured as scaffolds or multimeric constructs. Trimeric HIV-1 envelope glycoproteins, in particular, are likely to revolutionize the HIV vaccine field, as they will be able to identify trimer-specific mAbs, such as PGDM1400[52] and CAP256-VRC26 lineage antibodies. Multiple antibody lineages in one donor target the glycan-V3 supersite of the HIV-1 envelope glycoprotein and display a preference for quaternary binding,[40a] with remarkably specificity and efficiency. The production of stable soluble multimeric proteins, however, can be technically challenging and of limited generalizability to all antigen types. Some investigators have favored the display of antigens as membrane-bound structures on transformed cells or virus-like particles.[53–55] Although these constructs likely display the antigens in a relatively native conformation, without further processing, non native structures can also be displayed.[56] This, in turn, increases the chance of isolating antibodies of irrelevant specificity.

One way to enhance the specificity of isolated mAbs is to use multiple baits, where background signals are reduced by requiring binding to more than one reagent.[57] A stringent gating strategy for sorting on the flow cytometer can increase the likelihood that more specific mAbs are recovered, but potentially at the cost of losing B cells of interest. The optimal gating strategy, therefore, varies by the goals of the experiment, the technological capacity of the laboratory and the availability of samples and funds. Unfortunately, there are inherent problems that cannot be overcome by reagent choice alone, such as variable antibody expression levels on the surface of B cells and the fact that multimeric reagents can cause aggregation of cells during the experiment.[58] It remains to be seen if resolution of these problems results in an increased yield and specificity of isolated mAbs.

The development of new fluorochromes and conjugation techniques has steadily improved the overall utility of antigen reagents for screening B cells. There are three basic methods for labeling antibody baits: direct conjugation, binding to a prelabeled protein, and incorporation of a fluorochrome within the structure of the bait. The first method is straightforward as many conjugation kits are commercially available. However, conjugation is not specific to a particular region of the protein, carrying the potential of steric blockade or chemical alteration of the epitopes of interest. To overcome this problem, most investigators have transitioned to derivatization of bait reagents in a manner that is region specific. This is done by incorporating amino acid sequences that are specifically biotinylated. The bait can then either be used straight away after a streptavidin binding step in the cell staining procedure[59,60] or be prepared as a preformed reagent with streptavidin (i.e., B cell tetramer).[41] The latter technique is best suited when staining multiple fluorochromes to reduce background and can be used for the production of reagents that express differential epitopes (e.g., RSC3 and its derivatives). This technique has the added benefit of using fluorochromes that cannot be added by direct conjugation, either because of concerns about steric interference (e.g., allophycocyanin) or unavailability of commercial kits (e.g., brilliant violet dye series). Reagents can also be expressed as fusion proteins with a built-in fluorochrome, either as part of a particle or cell expressing the fluorochrome (e.g., green fluorescent protein) or in the context of a particle or cell that has been labeled by another technique (e.g., carboxyfluorescein succinimidyl ester). In each case, the choice of fluorochrome depends upon availability, machine configuration, ease of production and ability to be incorporated into the panel being used.

Investigators can also use the timing of immunologic events to increase the yield of antigen-specific B cells. For instance, plasmablasts specific for a particular antigen tend to be at their highest concentration at 7 days after vaccination.[21] The advantage of this technique is that it obviates the need for generating baits. However, it is less useful for the isolation of cells following diseases such as influenza,[3,20] where the majority of plasmablasts are not specific for the infecting pathogen. Still, plasma cell sorting can be useful when cell populations are limited (e.g., intestinal biopsies,[61] colostrum[62,63]) and the costs of personnel and laboratory supplies are prohibitive.

ISOLATION OF mABs BY NEXT-GENERATION SEQUENCING

Generation of functional monoclonal antibodies requires the identification of matched pairs of heavy and light chains. Recent advances in next-generation sequencing (NGS) of single B cells have opened up new possibilities for isolating new mAbs[64] (Fig. 1.1C). This approach probes unbiased plasmablast and memory B cell repertoires, generating thousands of paired sequences that are grouped into clonal families. Individual antibodies can then be expressed and screened through an intense selection process that employs the discipline of informatics. This process has been employed with some success for antibodies to HIV-1 and influenza. Interestingly, there is a much higher frequency of influenza-specific mAbs than HIV-specific mAbs in plasmablast populations from donors who have been infected with each pathogen.[3,65]

Unlike single cell sorting, the results of NGS do not depend on the amount of surface immunoglobulin present on a B cell. NGS technology also allows for the classification of antibodies by immunoglobulin subtype[66] and the molecular characterization of antibody classes. For example, the VRC01 class of CD4bs antibodies primarily derives from two variable heavy chain gene segments ($V_H1 \sim 2$ and $V_H1 \sim 46$).[41,67] Antibodies directed at the second variable loop (V2) of the HIV-1 gp120 envelope glycoprotein are typically isolated from HIV vaccine recipients and have a different amino acid motif in one of the complementarity determining region (CDR) loops.[68] Broadly neutralizing HIV-1 antibodies also have been well characterized and have exceptionally long CDR3 regions in their immunoglobulin heavy chains. These features have come as a direct result of a growing capability to mine large databases of antibody repertoires. However, antibodies identified through NGS still need to be expressed and functionally validated, limiting the actual numbers that can be tested. Additionally, the high level of antibody gene diversity in donors requires the careful selection of specific primers.[67] Despite these caveats, NGS technology is advancing rapidly and is becoming typified by increasing sequence read-lengths, reduced error-rates and more sophisticated bioinformatics tools for analysis.

TARGETS OF BROADLY NEUTRALIZING ANTIBODIES

The explosion in the number of new mAbs against HIV-1, influenza, RSV and other pathogens has enabled detailed antigenic and structural characterization of critical epitopes that are attractive targets for vaccine design. There are now hundreds of mAbs to the HIV-1 envelope glycoprotein that are classified into five major sites of neutralization: (1) CD4bs, (2) the V1/V2 loop, (3) the glycan rich V3 loop, (4) the gp120-gp41 interface, and (5) the MPER[69] (Fig. 1.2). While the neutralization capacity of a mAb against a specific region of the envelope glycoprotein varies across different HIV-1 subtypes, combinations of mAbs that target different epitopes can neutralize close to 100% of global isolates.[70] In the context of influenza, there is a broadly neutralizing class of antibodies that targets a conserved hydrophobic pocket in the membrane proximal region of the stem of the surface hemagglutinin (HA) glycoprotein. The prototype of this class, CR6261, was isolated from a recipient of seasonal influenza vaccine.[71] Subsequent structural analyses revealed that the antibody's binding was primarily mediated by residues in the heavy chain CDR1 and CDR2 that were encoded by germline genes.[72] A second class of influenza antibodies directed at the sialic acid receptor binding site on the HA has also been identified and is homologous to CD4bs antibodies to HIV-1. Several antibodies within this class have been described[73,74] and suggest that, unlike some HIV-1 antibodies[41,67] or the influenza HA stem antibodies,[71] this second class of antibodies is also derived from multiple germline genes.[75] Whether this will make it easier to design immunogens that elicit broadly neutralizing antibodies against influenza is still unknown.

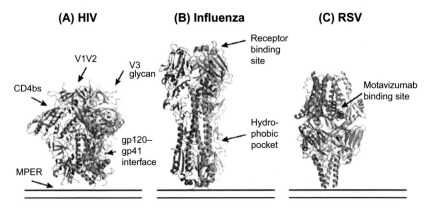

FIGURE 1.2 Broadly neutralizing antibody targets on (A) HIV, (B) Influenza, and (C) RSV. *Adapted from Pancera M, Zhou T, Druz A, Georgiev IS, Soto C, Gorman J, et al. Structure and immune recognition of trimeric pre-fusion HIV-1 Env. Nature. 2014;514(7523):455−61 [76].*

ISOLATION OF VACCINE-ELICITED mABs

Although a number of broadly neutralizing influenza-specific antibodies have been isolated from healthy vaccinated people, individuals who been vaccinated against HIV have generally yielded non-neutralizing mAbs.[77] Not surprisingly, these HIV-1 specific vaccine-elicited mAbs were considerably less mutated and had shorter heavy chain CDR3 regions compared to those from HIV-1 infected persons.[49] The most intensively studied HIV-1 vaccine trial to date, the ALVAC-prime AIDSVAX-boost RV144 trial[78] found two significant correlates of risk: low levels of IgG and high levels of IgA envelope binding antibodies.[79] With the aid of mAbs isolated from vaccine recipients, investigators were able to demonstrate a mechanism by which high levels of envelope-binding IgA could block the antibody-dependent cellular cytotoxicity (ADCC) activity of IgG antibodies directed at the same epitope.[80] The correlates analysis also found that the V1V2 loop of the envelope glycoprotein was a site of immune pressure[81] targeted by mAbs isolated from vaccine recipients.[51] A similar analysis showed that another site of immune pressure in gp120 V3 was also targeted by mAbs isolated from vaccine recipients.[82] Thus, the isolation of mAbs from vaccine recipients in the RV144 trial has resulted in a more detailed understanding of the mechanism of action responsible for the modest protection observed.

A subsequent vaccine trial, HVTN 505,[83] failed to demonstrate any protection against infection. While this immunization regimen was primarily designed to elicit T cell responses, it was the analysis of the B cell response that revealed critical new insights into mechanisms of immune diversion. Prior work on samples from HIV-1-infected individuals had shown that the earliest response to HIV-1 infection was directed against gp41,[84] that the plasmablast response in early HIV-1 infection was dominated by gp41-reactive antibodies[3] and that B cells resident in intestinal tissues were cross-reactive with gp41 and intestinal microbiota.[61] Isolation of mAbs from HVTN 505 vaccine recipients also demonstrated that the majority of the vaccine response was directed against gp41 but also was dominated by preexisting B cells that were cross-reactive with antigens from intestinal microbiota, and ultimately resulted in a non-protective response. Following the trend of these two examples, it is likely that future HIV-1 vaccine trials will be analyzed, at least in part, through the isolation of mAbs for the purpose of characterizing the B cell response. These analyses will enable a determination of whether desired responses are being subverted toward undesirable cross-reactivity. In addition, the study of efficacious vaccines, such as those against influenza, may offer guiding principles for the evaluation of novel vaccine candidates against currently circulating or novel pathogens.

mABs TARGETS IN VACCINE DESIGN

Reverse vaccinology and structure-based vaccine design relies on the principle that the target antigen of a protective mAb will elicit the same antibody response when used as an immunogen. Although this approach has taken time to bear fruit it has produced the meningococcal B vaccine for the prevention of *Neisseria meningitides*.[85] This approach can be further refined by using epitope-specific immunogens. For example, the engraftment of anti-RSV mAb motavizumab epitope onto a scaffolded protein has been shown to elicit neutralizing antibodies in animal models.[86] Although epitope-specific approaches toward vaccine design will need to be validated in humans they hold great promise for tackling other pathogens for which structural information of mAb targets is known. Unfortunately for HIV-1 no immunogens have yet been able to elicit broadly neutralizing antibody responses. This is probably in large part due to the complex nature of the HIV-1 glycoprotein which, until recently, has been difficult to reproduce in the laboratory.[87,88] Soluble native-like HIV-1 envelope trimers that display all the major neutralizing epitopes are now being tested in animals and shown to elicit better neutralizing responses than previous immunogens.[89]

USE OF mABs FOR THE PREVENTION AND TREATMENT OF INFECTIOUS DISEASES

The availability of an increasing number of broad and potent neutralizing antibodies has driven their use as both prophylactic and therapeutic products. Currently the only licensed anti-infective mAb is the recombinant Palivizumab (Synagis), which is injected monthly into newborn infants at high-risk for RSV infection.[90] However, passive immunization with polyclonal or convalescent sera has been in use for more than 100 years.[91] Thus for many diseases, the proof-of-principle of the protective role of serum antibodies already exists. In fact, a number of the important pathogens of the last century (i.e., measles, poliomyelitis) were first shown to be prevented with passive prophylaxis before active vaccines were developed. With the advent of increasingly efficient methods to isolate mAbs and growing knowledge about host-pathogen biology, the number of anti-infective mAbs with potential for clinical development is likely to expand significantly in the near future. A mAb cocktail for treatment of rabies infection has recently replaced polyclonal serum preparations[92] and mAbs shown to protect against Ebola infection in animals are being developed for human use.[93] A number of HIV-1 mAbs have recently entered human clinical trials, including the CD4bs mAbs 3BNC117 and VRC01,[94] with others that have shown efficacy in animal models coming along the pipeline.[95,96] For infections where no vaccines exist, such as HIV-1, the development of an immunoprophylaxis regimen could also help to answer important questions about minimal protective doses and relative efficacy of mAbs with different epitope-specificities and/or different isotypes. Furthermore, the ability of antibodies to bind and kill HIV-1 infected cells through Fc-mediated effector functions may make them players in a "shock and kill" cure strategy.[97] Interestingly, a mAb that targets the F protein of both RSV and MPV was found to require both effector and neutralizing function for protection but not for therapy.[15] This emphasizes the complex nature of the using biological reagents with underappreciated functions.

CONCLUSIONS

We are entering a new era in the prevention and treatment of infectious diseases, fueled by the isolation of functional mAbs that offer the promise of better vaccines and therapies (Fig. 1.3). Although the clinical use of anti-infective mAbs has lagged behind their use in cancers and inflammatory diseases, a surge in new mAbs coupled with advances in structural biology and computational vaccine design is likely to herald a new era for anti-pathogen mAbs. New mAbs against influenza, Ebola, RSV and HIV may result in improved vaccines and passive immunotherapy strategies. However, major obstacles still need to be overcome, particularly with regard to mAb mass production and cost. However, these barriers are being overcome with innovative advances in antibody manufacturing and delivery. In particular, new optimization strategies are enhancing the functional activity of mAbs and significantly extending their half-lives.[98] The expression of mAbs in adenovirus vectors has also enabled their sustained in vivo expression.[99] The isolation of mAbs from infected and vaccinated individuals has permitted rapid advances in our understanding of protective, and it is likely that their use

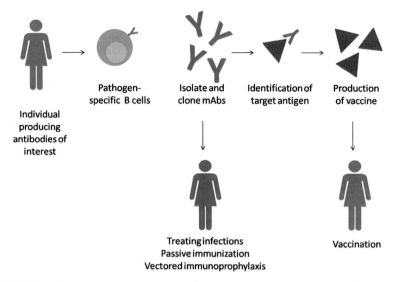

Individual producing antibodies of interest → Pathogen-specific B cells → Isolate and clone mAbs → Identification of target antigen → Production of vaccine

Treating infections
Passive immunization
Vectored immunoprophylaxis

Vaccination

FIGURE 1.3 How monoclonal antibodies are helping to design better treatments and vaccines.

will lead to broad applications in the fight against infectious diseases. It is our hope and expectation that mAbs will usher in an age of the iterative immunogen design that will accelerate the development of vaccines against otherwise intractable diseases.

ACKNOWLEDGMENTS

We would like to thank Dr. Carol Crowther for administrative assistance and Dr. Penny Moore and Dr. Nicole Doria-Rose for critical reading of the manuscript.

REFERENCES

1. Shlomchik MJ, Weisel F. Germinal center selection and the development of memory B and plasma cells. *Immunol Rev* 2012;**247**(1):52−63.
2. Pape KA, Taylor JJ, Maul RW, Gearhart PJ, Jenkins MK. Different B cell populations mediate early and late memory during an endogenous immune response. *Science* 2011;**331** (6021):1203−7.
3. Liao H-X, Chen X, Munshaw S, Zhang R, Marshall DJ, Vandergrift N, et al. Initial antibodies binding to HIV-1 gp41 in acutely infected subjects are polyreactive and highly mutated. *J Exp Med* 2011;**208**(11):2237−49.
4. Tonegawa S. Somatic generation of antibody diversity. *Nature* 1983;**302**(5909):575−81.
5. Di Noia JM, Neuberger MS. Molecular mechanisms of antibody somatic hypermutation. *Annu Rev Biochem* 2007;**76**:1−22.
6. Burton DR, Poignard P, Stanfield RL, Wilson IA. Broadly neutralizing antibodies present new prospects to counter highly antigenically diverse viruses. *Science* 2012;**337**(6091):183−6.

7. Plotkin SA. Complex correlates of protection after vaccination. *Clin Infect Dis* 2013;**56** (10):1458−65.

8. Simek MD, Rida W, Priddy FH, Pung P, Carrow E, Laufer DS, et al. Human immunodeficiency virus type 1 elite neutralizers: individuals with broad and potent neutralizing activity identified by using a high-throughput neutralization assay together with an analytical selection algorithm. *J Virol* 2009;**83**(14):7337−48.

9. Gray ES, Madiga MC, Hermanus T, Moore PL, Wibmer CK, Tumba NL, et al. The neutralization breadth of HIV-1 develops incrementally over four years and is associated with CD4$^+$ T cell decline and high viral load during acute infection. *J Virol* 2011;**85** (10):4828−40.

10. Doria-Rose NA, Klein RM, Daniels MG, O'Dell S, Nason M, Lapedes A, et al. Breadth of human immunodeficiency virus-specific neutralizing activity in sera: clustering analysis and association with clinical variables. *J Virol* 2010;**84**(3):1631−6.

11. van Gils MJ, Euler Z, Schweighardt B, Wrin T, Schuitemaker H. Prevalence of cross-reactive HIV-1-neutralizing activity in HIV-1-infected patients with rapid or slow disease progression. *AIDS* 2009;**23**(18):2405−14.

12. Sather DN, Armann J, Ching LK, Mavrantoni A, Sellhorn G, Caldwell Z, et al. Factors associated with the development of cross-reactive neutralizing antibodies during human immunodeficiency virus type 1 infection. *J Virol* 2009;**83**(2):757−69.

13. Klein F, Mouquet H, Dosenovic P, Scheid JF, Scharf L, Nussenzweig MC. Antibodies in HIV-1 vaccine development and therapy. *Science* 2013;**341**(6151):1199−204.

14. Burton DR, Mascola JR. Antibody responses to envelope glycoproteins in HIV-1 infection. *Nat Immunol* 2015;**16**(6):571−6.

15. Corti D, Bianchi S, Vanzetta F, Minola A, Perez L, Agatic G, et al. Cross-neutralization of four paramyxoviruses by a human monoclonal antibody. *Nature* 2013;**501**(7467):439−43.

16. Krause JC, Tsibane T, Tumpey TM, Huffman CJ, Albrecht R, Blum DL, et al. Human monoclonal antibodies to pandemic 1957 H2N2 and pandemic 1968 H3N2 influenza viruses. *J Virol* 2012;**86**(11):6334−40.

17. Wrammert J, Koutsonanos D, Li G-M, Edupuganti S, Sui J, Morrissey M, et al. Broadly cross-reactive antibodies dominate the human B cell response against 2009 pandemic H1N1 influenza virus infection. *J Exp Med* 2011;**208**(1):181−93.

18. Yu X, Tsibane T, McGraw PA, House FS, Keefer CJ, Hicar MD, et al. Neutralizing antibodies derived from the B cells of 1918 influenza pandemic survivors. *Nature* 2008;**455** (7212):532−6.

19. Corti D, Suguitan Jr. AL, Pinna D, Silacci C, Fernandez-Rodriguez BM, Vanzetta F, et al. Heterosubtypic neutralizing antibodies are produced by individuals immunized with a seasonal influenza vaccine. *J. Clin Invest* 2010;**120**(5):1663−73.

20. Moody MA, Zhang R, Walter EB, Woods CW, Ginsburg GS, McClain MT, et al. H3N2 influenza infection elicits more cross-reactive and less clonally expanded anti-hemagglutinin antibodies than influenza vaccination. *PloS One* 2011;**6**(10):e25797.

21. Wrammert J, Smith K, Miller J, Langley WA, Kokko K, Larsen C, et al. Rapid cloning of high-affinity human monoclonal antibodies against influenza virus. *Nature* 2008;**453** (7195):667−71.

22. Amanna IJ, Slifka MK. Mechanisms that determine plasma cell lifespan and the duration of humoral immunity. *Immunol Rev* 2010;**236**:125−38.

23. Stephenson KE, Neubauer GH, Reimer U, Pawlowski N, Knaute T, Zerweck J, et al. Quantification of the epitope diversity of HIV-1-specific binding antibodies by peptide microarrays for global HIV-1 vaccine development. *J Immunol Methods* 2015;**416**:105−23.

24. Tomaras GD, Binley JM, Gray ES, Crooks ET, Osawa K, Moore PL, et al. Polyclonal B cell responses to conserved neutralization epitopes in a subset of HIV-1-infected individuals. *J Virol* 2011;**85**(21):11502–19.

25. Binley JM, Lybarger EA, Crooks ET, Seaman MS, Gray E, Davis KL, et al. Profiling the specificity of neutralizing antibodies in a large panel of plasmas from patients chronically infected with human immunodeficiency virus type 1 subtypes B and C. *J Virol* 2008;**82**(23):11651–68.

26. Walker LM, Simek MD, Priddy F, Gach JS, Wagner D, Zwick MB, et al. A limited number of antibody specificities mediate broad and potent serum neutralization in selected HIV-1 infected individuals. *PLoS Pathog* 2010;**6**(8):e1001028.

27. Lynch RM, Tran L, Louder MK, Schmidt SD, Cohen M, Members CCT, et al. The development of CD4 binding site antibodies during HIV-1 infection. *J Virol* 2012;**86**(14):7588–95.

28. Li Y, Migueles SA, Welcher B, Svehla K, Phogat A, Louder MK, et al. Broad HIV-1 neutralization mediated by CD4-binding site antibodies. *Nat Med* 2007;**13**(9):1032–4.

29. Georgiev IS, Doria-Rose NA, Zhou T, Kwon YD, Staupe RP, Moquin S, et al. Delineating antibody recognition in polyclonal sera from patterns of HIV-1 isolate neutralization. *Science* 2013;**340**(6133):751–6.

30. Lacerda M, Moore PL, Ngandu NK, Seaman M, Gray ES, Murrell B, et al. Identification of broadly neutralizing antibody epitopes in the HIV-1 envelope glycoprotein using evolutionary models. *Virol J* 2013;**10**:347.

31. West Jr. AP, Scharf L, Horwitz J, Klein F, Nussenzweig MC, Bjorkman PJ. Computational analysis of anti-HIV-1 antibody neutralization panel data to identify potential functional epitope residues. *Proc Natl Acad Sci USA* 2013;**110**(26):10598–603.

32. Dejnirattisai W, Wongwiwat W, Supasa S, Zhang X, Dai X, Rouvinski A, et al. A new class of highly potent, broadly neutralizing antibodies isolated from viremic patients infected with dengue virus. *Nat Immunol* 2015;**16**(2):170–7.

33. Köhler G, Milstein C. Continuous cultures of fused cells secreting antibody of predefined specificity. *Nature* 1975;**256**(5517):495–7.

34. Corti D, Lanzavecchia A. Efficient methods to isolate human monoclonal antibodies from memory B cells and plasma cells. *Microbiol Spectr* 2014;**2**:5.

35. Roberts ML, Luxembourg AT, Cooper NR. Epstein-Barr virus binding to CD21, the virus receptor, activates resting B cells via an intracellular pathway that is linked to B cell infection. *J Gen Virol* 1996;**77**(Pt 12):3077–85.

36. Bonsignori M, Hwang K-K, Chen X, Tsao C-Y, Morris L, Gray E, et al. Analysis of a clonal lineage of HIV-1 envelope V2/V3 conformational epitope-specific broadly neutralizing antibodies and their inferred unmutated common ancestors. *J Virol* 2011;**85**(19):9998–10009.

37. Walker LM, Phogat SK, Chan-Hui PY, Wagner D, Phung P, Goss JL, et al. Broad and potent neutralizing antibodies from an African donor reveal a new HIV-1 vaccine target. *Science* 2009;**326**(5950):285–9.

38. Huang J, Doria-Rose NA, Longo NS, Laub L, Lin CL, Turk E, et al. Isolation of human monoclonal antibodies from peripheral blood B cells. *Nat Protoc* 2013;**8**(10):1907–15.

39. Walker LM, Huber M, Doores KJ, Falkowska E, Pejchal R, Julien JP, et al. Broad neutralization coverage of HIV by multiple highly potent antibodies. *Nature* 2011;**477**(7365):466–70.

40. Avery DT, Bryant VL, Ma CS, de Waal Malefyt R, Tangye SG. IL-21-induced isotype switching to IgG and IgA by human naive B cells is differentially regulated by IL-4. *J Immunol* 2008;**181**(3):1767–79.

40a. Longo NS, Sutton MS, Shiakolas AR, Guenaga J, Jarosinski MC, Georgiev IS, et al. Multiple antibody lineages in one donor target the glycan-V3 supersite of the HIV-1 envelope glycoprotein and display a preference for quaternary binding. *J Virol.* 2016 Sep 21. pii: JVI.01012-16. [Epub ahead of print] PMID: 27654288.

41. Wu X, Yang ZY, Li Y, Hogerkorp CM, Schief WR, Seaman MS, et al. Rational design of envelope identifies broadly neutralizing human monoclonal antibodies to HIV-1. *Science* 2010;**329**(5993):856−61.

42. Zhou T, Lynch RM, Chen L, Acharya P, Wu X, Doria-Rose NA, et al. Structural repertoire of HIV-1-neutralizing antibodies targeting the CD4 supersite in 14 donors. *Cell* 2015;**161** (6):1280−92.

43. Newman J, Rice JS, Wang C, Harris SL, Diamond B. Identification of an antigen-specific B cell population. *J Immunol Methods* 2003;**272**(1−2):177−87.

44. Morris L, Chen X, Alam M, Tomaras G, Zhang R, Marshall DJ, et al. Isolation of a human anti-HIV gp41 membrane proximal region neutralizing antibody by antigen-specific single B cell sorting. *PloS One* 2011;**6**(9):e23532.

45. Holl TM, Yang G, Kuraoka M, Verkoczy L, Alam SM, Moody MA, et al. *Enhanced antibody responses to an HIV-1 membrane-proximal external region antigen in mice reconstituted with cultured lymphocytes* 2014;**192**(7):3269−79.

46. Verkoczy L, Moody MA, Holl TM, Bouton-Verville H, Scearce RM, Hutchinson J, et al. Functional, non-clonal IgMa-restricted B cell receptor interactions with the HIV-1 envelope gp41 membrane proximal external region. *PLoS One* 2009;**4**(10):e7215.

47. Yang G, Holl TM, Liu Y, Li Y, Lu X, Nicely NI, et al. Identification of autoantigens recognized by the 2F5 and 4E10 broadly neutralizing HIV-1 antibodies. *J Exp Med* 2013;**210** (2):241−56.

48. Gray ES, Moody MA, Wibmer CK, Chen X, Marshall D, Amos J, et al. Isolation of a monoclonal antibody that targets the alpha-2 helix of gp120 and represents the initial autologous neutralizing-antibody response in an HIV-1 subtype C-infected individual. *J Virol* 2011;**85**(15):7719−29.

49. Bonsignori M, Pollara J, Moody MA, Alpert MD, Chen X, Hwang K-K, et al. Antibody-dependent cellular cytotoxicity-mediating antibodies from an HIV-1 vaccine efficacy trial target multiple epitopes and preferentially use the VH1 gene family. *J Virol* 2012;**86** (21):11521−32.

50. Moody MA, Yates NL, Amos JD, Drinker MS, Eudailey JA, Gurley TC, et al. HIV-1 gp120 vaccine induces affinity maturation in both new and persistent antibody clonal lineages. *J Virol* 2012;**86**(14):7496−507.

51. Liao HX, Bonsignori M, Alam SM, McLellan JS, Tomaras GD, Moody MA, et al. Vaccine induction of antibodies against a structurally heterogeneous site of immune pressure within HIV-1 envelope protein variable regions 1 and 2. *Immunity* 2013;**38**(1):176−86.

52. Sok D, van Gils MJ, Pauthner M, Julien JP, Saye-Francisco KL, Hsueh J, et al. Recombinant HIV envelope trimer selects for quaternary-dependent antibodies targeting the trimer apex. *Proc Natl Acad Sci USA* 2014;**111**(49):17624−9.

53. Hicar MD, Chen X, Briney B, Hammonds J, Wang J-J, Kalams S, et al. Pseudovirion particles bearing native HIV envelope trimers facilitate a novel method for generating human neutralizing monoclonal antibodies against HIV. *JAIDS J Acquir Immune Defic Syndr* 2010;**54**(3):223−35.

54. Hicar MD, Kalams SA, Spearman PW, Crowe Jr. JE. Emerging studies of human HIV-specific antibody repertoires. *Vaccine* 2010;**28**(Suppl. 2):B18−23.

55. Klein F, Gaebler C, Mouquet H, Sather DN, Lehmann C, Scheid JF, et al. Broad neutralization by a combination of antibodies recognizing the CD4 binding site and a new conformational epitope on the HIV-1 envelope protein. *J Exp Med* 2012;**209**(8):1469−79.

56. Crooks ET, Tong T, Osawa K, Binley JM. Enzyme digests eliminate nonfunctional Env from HIV-1 particle surfaces, leaving native Env trimers intact and viral infectivity unaffected. *J Virol* 2011;**85**(12):5825−39.

57. Kodituwakku AP, Jessup C, Zola H, Roberton DM. Isolation of antigen-specific B cells. *Immunol Cell Biol* 2003;**81**(3):163–70.

58. Moody MA, Haynes BF. Antigen-specific B cell detection reagents: use and quality control. *Cytometry Part A* 2008;**73**(11):1086–92.

59. Doria-Rose NA, Klein RM, Manion MM, O'Dell S, Phogat A, Chakrabarti B, et al. Frequency and phenotype of human immunodeficiency virus envelope-specific B cells from patients with broadly cross-neutralizing antibodies. *J Virol* 2009;**83**(1):188–99.

60. Scheid JF, Mouquet H, Feldhahn N, Walker BD, Pereyra F, Cutrell E, et al. A method for identification of HIV gp140 binding memory B cells in human blood. *J Immunol Methods* 2009;**343**(2):65–7.

61. Trama AM, Moody MA, Alam SM, Jaeger FH, Lockwood B, Parks R, et al. HIV-1 envelope gp41 antibodies can originate from terminal ileum B cells that share cross-reactivity with commensal bacteria. *Cell Host Microbe* 2014;**16**(2):215–26.

62. Friedman J, Alam SM, Shen X, Xia S-M, Stewart S, Anasti K, et al. Isolation of HIV-1-neutralizing mucosal monoclonal antibodies from human colostrum. *PLoS One* 2012;**7**(5): e37648.

63. Sacha CR, Vandergrift N, Jeffries TL, McGuire E, Fouda GG, Liebl B, et al. Restricted isotype, distinct variable gene usage, and high rate of gp120 specificity of HIV-1 envelope-specific B cells in colostrum compared with those in blood of HIV-1-infected, lactating African women. *Mucosal Immunol* 2015;**8**(2):316–26.

64. DeKosky BJ, Ippolito GC, Deschner RP, Lavinder JJ, Wine Y, Rawlings BM, et al. High-throughput sequencing of the paired human immunoglobulin heavy and light chain repertoire. *Nat Biotechnol* 2013;**31**(2):166–9.

65. Jackson KJ, Liu Y, Roskin KM, Glanville J, Hoh RA, Seo K, et al. Human responses to influenza vaccination show seroconversion signatures and convergent antibody rearrangements. *Cell Host Microbe* 2014;**16**(1):105–14.

66. Schanz M, Liechti T, Zagordi O, Miho E, Reddy ST, Gunthard HF, et al. High-throughput sequencing of human immunoglobulin variable regions with subtype identification. *PLoS One* 2014;**9**(11):e111726.

67. Scheid JF, Mouquet H, Ueberheide B, Diskin R, Klein F, Oliveira TY, et al. Sequence and structural convergence of broad and potent HIV antibodies that mimic CD4 binding. *Science* 2011;**333**(6049):1633–7.

68. Wiehe K, Easterhoff D, Luo K, Nicely NI, Bradley T, Jaeger FH, et al. Antibody light-chain-restricted recognition of the site of immune pressure in the RV144 HIV-1 vaccine trial is phylogenetically conserved. *Immunity* 2014;**41**(6):909–18.

69. Wibmer CK, Moore PL, Morris L. HIV broadly neutralizing antibody targets. *Curr Opin HIV AIDS* 2015;**10**(3):135–43.

70. Kong R, Louder MK, Wagh K, Bailer RT, deCamp A, Greene K, et al. Improving neutralization potency and breadth by combining broadly reactive HIV-1 antibodies targeting major neutralization epitopes. *J Virol* 2015;**89**(5):2659–71.

71. Throsby M, van den Brink E, Jongeneelen M, Poon LLM, Alard P, Cornelissen L, et al. Heterosubtypic neutralizing monoclonal antibodies cross-protective against H5N1 and H1N1 recovered from human IgM + memory B cells. *PLoS One* 2008;**3**(12):e3942.

72. Ekiert DC, Bhabha G, Elsliger M-A, Friesen RHE, Jongeneelen M, Throsby M, et al. Antibody recognition of a highly conserved influenza virus epitope. *Science* 2009;**324** (5924):246–51.

73. Whittle JR, Zhang R, Khurana S, King LR, Manischewitz J, Golding H, et al. Broadly neutralizing human antibody that recognizes the receptor-binding pocket of influenza virus hemagglutinin. *Proc Natl Acad Sci USA* 2011;**108**(34):14216–21.

74. Hong M, Lee PS, Hoffman RM, Zhu X, Krause JC, Laursen NS, et al. Antibody recognition of the pandemic H1N1 Influenza virus hemagglutinin receptor binding site. *J Virol* 2013;**87**(22):12471−80.

75. Schmidt AG, Therkelsen MD, Stewart S, Kepler TB, Liao HX, Moody MA, et al. Viral receptor-binding site antibodies with diverse germline origins. *Cell* 2015;**161**(5):1026−34.

76. Pancera M, Zhou T, Druz A, Georgiev IS, Soto C, Gorman J, et al. Structure and immune recognition of trimeric pre-fusion HIV-1 Env. *Nature* 2014;**514**(7523):455−61.

77. Montefiori DC, Karnasuta C, Huang Y, Ahmed H, Gilbert P, de Souza MS, et al. Magnitude and breadth of the neutralizing antibody response in the RV144 and Vax003 HIV-1 vaccine efficacy trials. *J Infect Dis* 2012;**206**(3):431−41.

78. Rerks-Ngarm S, Pitisuttithum P, Nitayaphan S, Kaewkungwal J, Chiu J, Paris R, et al. Vaccination with ALVAC and AIDSVAX to prevent HIV-1 infection in Thailand. *N Engl J Med* 2009;**361**(23):2209−20.

79. Haynes BF, Gilbert PB, McElrath MJ, Zolla-Pazner S, Tomaras GD, Alam SM, et al. Immune-correlates analysis of an HIV-1 vaccine efficacy trial. *N Engl J Med* 2012;**366** (14):1275−86.

80. Tomaras GD, Ferrari G, Shen X, Alam SM, Liao HX, Pollara J, et al. Vaccine-induced plasma IgA specific for the C1 region of the HIV-1 envelope blocks binding and effector function of IgG. *Proc Natl Acad Sci USA* 2013;**110**(22):9019−24.

81. Rolland M, Edlefsen PT, Larsen BB, Tovanabutra S, Sanders-Buell E, Hertz T, et al. Increased HIV-1 vaccine efficacy against viruses with genetic signatures in Env V2. *Nature* 2012;**490**(7420):417−20.

82. Zolla-Pazner S, Edlefsen PT, Rolland M, Kong XP, deCamp A, Gottardo R, et al. Vaccine-induced human antibodies specific for the third variable region of HIV-1 gp120 impose immune pressure on infecting viruses. *EBioMedicine* 2014;**1**(1):37−45.

83. Hammer SM, Sobieszczyk ME, Janes H, Karuna ST, Mulligan MJ, Grove D, et al. Efficacy trial of a DNA/rAd5 HIV-1 preventive vaccine. *N Engl J Med.* 2013;**369** (22):2083−92.

84. Tomaras GD, Yates NL, Liu P, Qin L, Fouda GG, Chavez LL, et al. Initial B-cell responses to transmitted human immunodeficiency virus type 1: virion-binding immunoglobulin M (IgM) and IgG antibodies followed by plasma anti-gp41 antibodies with ineffective control of initial viremia. *J Virol* 2008;**82**(24):12449−63.

85. Oviedo-Orta E, Ahmed S, Rappuoli R, Black S. Prevention and control of meningococcal outbreaks: the emerging role of serogroup B meningococcal vaccines. *Vaccine* 2015;**33** (31):3628−35.

86. Correia BE, Bates JT, Loomis RJ, Baneyx G, Carrico C, Jardine JG, et al. Proof of principle for epitope-focused vaccine design. *Nature* 2014;**507**(7491):201−6.

87. Lyumkis D, Julien JP, de Val N, Cupo A, Potter CS, Klasse PJ, et al. Cryo-EM structure of a fully glycosylated soluble cleaved HIV-1 envelope trimer. *Science* 2013;**342**(6165):1484−90.

88. Julien JP, Cupo A, Sok D, Stanfield RL, Lyumkis D, Deller MC, et al. Crystal structure of a soluble cleaved HIV-1 envelope trimer. *Science* 2013;**342**(6165):1477−83.

89. Sanders RW, van Gils MJ, Derking R, Sok D, Ketas TJ, Burger JA, et al. HIV-1 neutralizing antibodies induced by native-like envelope trimers. *Science* 2015;**349**(6244):aac4223.

90. Palivizumab, a humanized respiratory syncytial virus monoclonal antibody, reduces hospitalization from respiratory syncytial virus infection in high-risk infants. Pediatrics. 1998;102(3).531−7.

91. Graham BS, Ambrosino DM. History of passive antibody administration for prevention and treatment of infectious diseases. *Curr Opin HIV AIDS* 2015;**10**(3):129−34.

92. Both L, Banyard AC, van Dolleweerd C, Horton DL, Ma JK, Fooks AR. Passive immunity in the prevention of rabies. *Lancet Infect Dis* 2012;**12**(5):397−407.

93. Qiu X, Wong G, Audet J, Bello A, Fernando L, Alimonti JB, et al. Reversion of advanced Ebola virus disease in nonhuman primates with ZMapp. *Nature* 2014;**514**(7520):47−53.

94. Caskey M, Klein F, Lorenzi JC, Seaman MS, West Jr. AP, Buckley N, et al. Viraemia suppressed in HIV-1-infected humans by broadly neutralizing antibody 3BNC117. *Nature* 2015;**522**(7557):487−91.

95. Shingai M, Nishimura Y, Klein F, Mouquet H, Donau OK, Plishka R, et al. Antibody-mediated immunotherapy of macaques chronically infected with SHIV suppresses viraemia. *Nature* 2013;**503**(7475):277−80.

96. Barouch DH, Whitney JB, Moldt B, Klein F, Oliveira TY, Liu J, et al. Therapeutic efficacy of potent neutralizing HIV-1-specific monoclonal antibodies in SHIV-infected rhesus monkeys. *Nature* 2013;**503**(7475):224−8.

97. Euler Z, Alter G. Exploring the potential of monoclonal antibody therapeutics for HIV-1 eradication. *AIDS Res Hum Retroviruses* 2015;**31**(1):13−24.

98. Sievers SA, Scharf L, West Jr. AP, Bjorkman PJ. Antibody engineering for increased potency, breadth and half-life. *Curr Opin HIV AIDS* 2015;**10**(3):151−9.

99. Balazs AB, Chen J, Hong CM, Rao DS, Yang L, Baltimore D. Antibody-based protection against HIV infection by vectored immunoprophylaxis. *Nature* 2012;**481**(7379):81−4.

Part II

Pathogen Free Vaccines

Chapter 2

Replication-Competent Viral Vectors for Vaccine Delivery

C.L. Parks
The International AIDS Vaccine Initiative, Brooklyn, NY, United States

INTRODUCTION

The development of a safe and effective vaccine is a long and challenging process, irrespective of the target pathogen. This is particularly true for human immunodeficiency virus (HIV), where there have been both unique and prototypical obstacles to creating vaccine delivery technologies that elicit sufficient acquired immunity to prevent or abort HIV infection, or control viral replication. To date, few candidate HIV vaccines have been tested in efficacy trials,[1−4] limiting the number of delivery technologies that have been subjected to this rigorous assessment. In four efficacy trials, delivery vectors based on replication-defective viruses were evaluated as part of the vaccination regimen. Limited efficacy was observed in the RV144 clinical trial in which host-restricted canarypox vectors (ALVAC) encoding Gag, Pro, and Env were used in combination with Env subunit vaccines.[3,5,6] Efficacy was not observed in three other trials where replication-defective adenovirus type 5 (Ad5) vectors were used: HVTN 502 (Step trial), HVTN 503 (Phambili trial), and HVTN 505 (DNA/Ad5).[7−9] Although efficacy was limited in the RV144 trial, and the regimens incorporating Ad5 failed to generate protective immunity, it is important to highlight that the nonreplicating viral vectors were components of vaccination regimens that effectively evoked immune responses in trial volunteers. Thus these results supported continued investigation of viral vector delivery technologies, but also showed that vector design changes were essential to elicit durable protective immunity.

Why investigate replicating vectors? One of the most compelling reasons for investigating replicating viral vectors comes from the historical success of vaccination programs in which live attenuated viral vaccines (LAVVs) were used safely to control the spread of disease caused by highly infectious

Human Vaccines: Emerging Technologies in Design and Development.
DOI: http://dx.doi.org/10.1016/B978-0-12-802302-0.00001-7

human and animal pathogens (Table 2.1).[12–14] The mild or subclinical infection caused by LAVVs is very effective at generating immunity that prevents disease and subsequent transmission. The LAVV approach used for licensed products, such as the measles, polio and yellow fever vaccines, also has been applied to experimental models such as simian acquired immunodeficiency syndrome (AIDS) in rhesus macaques. Immunity induced in macaques by infection with attenuated strains of SIV, such as SIVmac239Δnef, protects animals from rapid disease progression caused by infection with highly

TABLE 2.1 Listing of Live Attenuated Viral Vaccines Currently or Formerly Used in the United States

Live Attenuated Viral Vaccines for Human Diseases

Disease	Virus	Family	Route of Vaccination
DNA			
Smallpox[a]	Variola	Poxvirus	Scarification
Varicella	Varicellazoster virus	Herpesvirus	Subcutaneous
Acute respiratory/ enteric illness	Adenovirus 4/7	Adenovirus	**Oral capsule**
Positive Strand RNA			
Poliomyelitis & paralytic polio[b]	Polio virus	Picornavirus	**Oral liquid**
Yellow fever	Yellow fever virus	Flavivirus	Intramuscular
Rubella & congenital rubella syndrome	Rubella virus	Togavirus	Subcutaneous
Double-Stranded RNA			
Acute viral gastroenteritis	Rotavirus	Reovirus	**Oral solution**
Negative Strand RNA			
Measles	Measles virus	Paramyxovirus	Subcutaneous
Mumps	Mumps virus	Paramyxovirus	Subcutaneous
Influenza	Influenza virus	Orthomyxovirus	**Intranasal spray**

Several mucosal delivery routes are emphasized in bold text; additional information about the content of the table can be found in other sources.[21,22]
[a]Disease has been eradicated using live attenuated vaccines.[23]
[b]Use of the inactivated poliovirus has superseded the live attenuated vaccine in some countries.[24]

virulent challenge virus like SIVmac239.[15,16] Further studies also showed that protection conferred by live attenuated SIV is dependent on replicative capacity, as more attenuated variants do not elicit the same degree of protective immunity.[17−19] The importance of replicative capacity in generating immunity against SIV may also extend to vectors, as illustrated by studies showing that vaccination with replication-defective Ad5-SIV vaccines only has a modest inhibitory effect on SIVmac239 replication in infected macaques.[16,20]

The proven efficacy of licensed LAVVs and the immune protection provided by SIVmac239Δnef in macaques suggests that a vaccine based on live attenuated HIV could prove to be effective. However, using a live lentivirus as a vaccine in humans is impractical because there are significant risks associated with genome integration, viral genome recombination and genetic reversion that could results in chronic infection and disease.[25] Thus, for HIV, as well as some other highly virulent pathogens, replication-competent vectors offer a safer alternative platform for generating immunity equivalent to that elicited by live attenuated viruses.[26]

REPLICATING VECTOR DESIGNS

Adenovirus serotype 5 (Ad5) was one of the earliest viruses that could be genetically manipulated.[27,28] Since then, other viral genetic manipulation systems have emerged, making it possible to investigate viral vectors with considerably different biological properties or technical advantages. This expanding portfolio of viral vector platforms, including those based on replication-competent viruses, provides important advantages for vaccine development. In the context of HIV vaccines, vectors could be designed to mimic specific properties of the protective live attenuated SIVmac239Δnef vaccine. For example, there has been some focus on creating viral vectors that deliver various constructs of the envelope protein (Env) displayed on virus particles that range from discrete epitopes to authentic membrane-bound trimeric spikes, as occurs during an SIV or HIV infection. There also has been investigation of vectors that can establish a persistent infection, infect lymphoid tissues, or both, as does live attenuated SIV. Other important factors that have influenced vector selection and development include their prospective use for mucosal vaccine delivery, and their potential to minimize possible effects of preexisting anti-vector immunity. The vector descriptions below highlight some of the unique design features and biological properties that are being applied to vaccine vector development, with a particular focus on HIV vaccine candidates. The descriptions in the text are not comprehensive of all replicating viral vectors under investigation. Additional vectors can be found in Table 2.2, other review articles[26,29−38] and a growing publicly available database.[39]

Additional citations are included in the text.

TABLE 2.2 Listing of Replicating Viral Vectors Being Investigated as SIV or HIV Vaccines

Vector	Development Stage	Literature Citation or Clinical Trial Information
DNA Viruses		
Human adenovirus type 4	Preclinical/clinical development	40,41 NCT01989533
Human adenovirus type 5	NHP	42−44
Human adenovirus type 26	Clinical Development	45,46 NCT02366013
Simian adenovirus	Preclinical development	47
Rhesus cytomegalovirus	NHP	48,49
Human cytomegalovirus	Preclinical / clinical development	L. Picker, in progress
Herpes simplex virus	NHP	50
Rhesus rhadinovirus	NHP	51
Varicella zoster virus	NHP	52
Vaccinia virus—Tiantan	Clinical trial, ClinicalTrials.gov	35,53 NCT01705223
Vaccina virus—NYVAC-KC	NHP	54,55
Vaccinia virus—modified Tiantan	Preclinical development	56
Vaccinia virus—Guang9	Preclinical development	57
Vaccinia virus—LC16m8	Preclinical development	58
RNA Virus—Positive Strand		
Coxsackie virus	Preclinical development	59
Poliovirus	NHP	60,61
Rubella virus	Preclinical development	62
Semliki Forrest virus chimeras	NHP	63,64
Venezuelan equine encephalitis virus chimeras	NHP	65
Yellow fever virus	NHP	66,67

(Continued)

TABLE 2.2 (Continued)

Vector	Development Stage	Literature Citation or Clinical Trial Information
RNA Virus—Double Strand		
Reovirus	Preclinical	68
RNA Virus—Negative Strand		
Canine distemper virus	NHP	69
Influenza virus	Preclinical and NHP	70,71
Measles virus	Clinical trial	72,73 NCT01320176
Measles virus chimeras	Preclinical development	74
Mumps virus	Preclinical development	75
Newcastle disease virus	Preclinical development	76—78
Rabies virus	NHP	79,80
Parainfluenza virus-Sendai virus	NHP and Clinical Trial	81,82 NCT01705990
Parainfluenza virus—PIV5	NHP	83
Vesicular stomatitis virus	Clinical trial	84—87 NCT01578889
Vesicular stomatitis virus chimeras	NHP	88,89

Some vectors not described in the text are included here. *NHP,* nonhuman primate studies. Additional citations are included in the text.

DNA VIRUS VECTORS

The adenoviruses (Ads), herpesviruses, and poxviruses each have unique features that make them important platforms for development and investigation of replication-competent vectors. Intensive evaluation of replication-defective Ad vectors has shown them to be effective for gene delivery. Ads naturally infect the respiratory and gastrointestinal tract of humans and animals, suggesting that replication-competent variants would be valuable to investigate as mucosal delivery vectors.[90,91] The herpesviruses establish a life-long infection, and accordingly, they are one of the few viruses that can be used as a vector that will drive long-term antigen expression and immune stimulation[36] without modifying the host genome. Poxvirus vectors, best exemplified by the host-restricted canarypox ALVAC-HIV vaccine, were immunogenic in RV144 clinical trial,[3] suggesting potential gains in immunogenicity or immune response durability might be achieved with related replication-competent poxvirus vectors.

Adenoviruses

Replication-defective Ad5 vectors have been shown to be effective at stimulating CD8T cell responses in clinical trials.[92,93] These replication-defective vectors showed lack of efficacy and, in one case, an increase in HIV acquisition in a sub-population with existing Ad5 immunity.[94,95] Consequently, research and development priorities shifted to alternative human or simian Ad vectors[96–100] to which there is a lower prevalence of preexisting immunity. In some cases, these alternative Ad vectors, some of which are being developed as replication competent antigen delivery vehicles,[40,45,101] use different cellular receptors that change cell tropism and signaling pathways that are triggered by virus attachment.[102]

In general, the replication-competent Ad vectors differ from their replication-defective counterparts by the presence of Early Region 1 (E1; Fig. 2.1). E1 encodes polypeptides that are important for autonomous

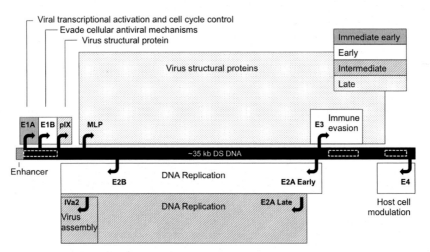

FIGURE 2.1 Summary of adenovirus transcription units. Transcription units are shown along with some of the functions associated with the proteins expressed from the different gene regions.[10,11] The double stranded DNA genome (black) is transcribed on both strands. The boundaries of sequences that are frequently deleted to make room for foreign inserts are shown as boxes drawn with white dashed lines. Timing of transcription unit activity is shaded according to the key at the top right. E1a is transcribed first due to the activity of the *cis*-acting enhancer sequence in the left end of the genome. One of the polypeptides encoded by E1a subsequently activates transcription of the early promoters. The intermediate promoters are activated at the onset of DNA replication and the major late promoter (MLP) transcription unit becomes fully active later as DNA synthesis progresses.

replication, blocking host interferon responses, and preventing premature cell death.[103,104] The inclusion of E1 in the viral vector genome provides autonomous replicative capacity but also takes up genomic space commonly used for foreign gene inserts. Due to the fact that the symmetrical Ad capsid has relatively strict upper size limits for packaged DNA,[105] deletion of DNA sequences at other sites in the genome is required to make room for foreign genes, and typically, deletions are made in the E3 and E4 genes, which encode multiple proteins that play important roles in immune evasion, such as down-regulation of MHC Class I expression (E3) and inactivation of the intracellular antiviral response (E4).[106−108] Consequently, replication-competent Ad vectors likely will be attenuated in vivo and their interaction with the innate and adaptive immune system will be modulated by the specific E3 and E4 modifications introduced during vector construction.[45,109] How this will affect B and T cell responses elicited by a replication-competent Ad vector will need to be established empirically.

Several different replicating Ad vectors are being developed primarily for mucosal vaccine delivery. Replication-competent Ad4 and Ad7 vectors delivered in enteric capsules have been used to vaccinate military personnel against respiratory and gastrointestinal illness since the 1970s,[110,111] and now Ad4 is in development as a replicating vector as well. A replicating Ad4 vector was safely tested in a recent clinical trial,[41] in which it effectively primed antibody responses against influenza virus hemagglutinin (H5). Ad4 encoding HIV Env (clade C.1086) also has been shown to elicit antibodies in rabbits vaccinated via intramuscular or intranasal administration.[40] Vectors encoding HIV Gag and Env antigens delivered by oral capsule or intranasal solution are presently being evaluated in a phase I clinical trial (ClinicalTrials.gov NCT01989533).

Replication-defective Ad26 has been assessed in nonhuman primates[112−114] and in phase I trials,[115−117] and more recently, replication-competent variants containing the Ad E1 region have been developed.[45] Preclinical assessment of replication-competent Ad26-Env vectors showed that they could be safely administered to mice by intramuscular injection or by intranasal instillation, and that both vaccination routes elicited antibodies. A replication-competent Ad26-based vaccine for oral administration has been developed and will be tested in a phase I trial (ClinicalTrial.gov NCT02366013).

Two other Ad serotypes are being investigated as replicating vectors. Preclinical assessment of replication-competent Ad5 continues, as it can be delivered mucosally.[32] As part of different prime-boost regimens, replicating Ad5 vectors delivering SIV genes have elicited mucosal and non-mucosal immune responses shown to be effective against SIVmac251.[42,43,101] Ad6 vectors that encode the E1 polypeptides, and are either replication-competent or have a capsid mutation that limits replication to a single round,[118] have been evaluated in preclinical studies conducted in hamsters and macaques. Interestingly, increased antibody responses were evoked by the vector containing the capsid mutation compared to a replication-competent version of the vector. The enhanced antibody response elicited by the single-cycle vector may be due to the non-propagating variant being able to persist for a greater period of time, or because it generates a different innate response signature compared to the replication-competent counterpart.[118]

As the HVTN 502 STEP trial indicated that there was increased HIV infection in a subgroup of people who had been vaccinated with replication-defective Ad5-HIV,[119] subsequent development of Ad vectors have raised questions about their potential to activate CD4 cells.[120] Studies in the rhesus macaque model also point to replication-defective Ad5 vectors causing increased homing of activated CD4 cells to the gut lymphoid tissue.[121,122] As these results were generated with replication-defective Ad vectors, it will be important to learn whether replication-competent vaccines containing an intact E1 region and various deletions in E3 or E4 yield a similar profile of immune responses. It will also be important to understand the immunologic impact of modifications to newer Ad vectors that are based on alternative serotypes that have different receptor usage, cell and tissue tropism, and route of administration (mucosal vs intramuscular),[91,100] as it is likely that some of the new Ad-based vaccine regimens will generate a different profile of immunity.

Poxviruses

Poxviruses that can infect human cells but undergo an abortive infection have been studied widely as vaccine vectors, such as host-restricted vaccinia virus strains like modified vaccinia Ankara (MVA) or NYVAC, and avipoxviruses (fowlpox and canarypox).[123−126] Interest remains high in continuing the development nonreplicating poxvirus vectors, as they can be used safely in humans and because a canarypox vector was used in the RV-144 clinical trial.[3,5] However, vaccinia virus vectors with increased replicative capacity also are being developed to deliver HIV genes. The most advanced is based on the vaccinia virus Tiantan (VTT) strain, present in a Chinese smallpox vaccine A.[127] A VVT-HIV vaccine delivered by scarification caused skin reactions typical of smallpox vaccination and induced HIV-specific T cell responses in vaccinia virus-naïve human trial participants.[35,53,128] A phase II study with VVT-HIV has been completed (National Center for AIDS/STD Control and Prevention, China CDC; ClinicalTrials.gov NCT01705223), where it was used as a boost for a DNA prime administered by electroporation.[128] In preclinical studies, VTT encoding SIV Gag and HIV Env also was shown to induce neutralizing antibodies active against an autologous simian-human immunodeficiency virus (SHIV) challenge in Chinese rhesus macaques.[129]

Although some of the genes will vary in different vectors, poxviruses encode a number of polypeptides dedicated to modulating the host cell environment and immune response to infection.[130,131] Manipulation of these genes has proven to be a useful strategy for generating vectors that vary in their immunostimulatory properties as well as their performance in murine models. A modified VVT (MVVT), in which several genes have been deleted, has been shown to elicit immunity that provided significant protection in Chinese rhesus macaques challenged with SIVmac239 when immunization was conducted with a mucosal MVVT-SIV prime and intramuscular Ad5-SIV boost regimen.[56,132,133] The vaccinia virus strain NYVAC,[134] which normally undergoes an abortive infection in human cells, has been modified by systematically adding genes to restore replicative capacity to varying degrees.[54,55] The replication-competent NYVAC-KC vectors have been tested safely in macaques[135] and were found to be more potent inducers of cellular and humoral immunity when compared to nonreplicating NYVAC vectors.[136]

Herpesviruses

Herpesviruses are large-enveloped DNA viruses that have evolved immune evasion mechanisms that enable them to establish life-long infections.[137] Since they do establish long-term virus host-interactions, several herpesviruses are being investigated as vectors to provide persistent T cell stimulation that duplicates the protective effect observed in macaques that are infected with live attenuated SIV. Moreover, herpesviruses might also prove useful as HIV Env delivery vectors, because of their potential to provide long-term immunogen exposure needed to help drive emergence of antibodies with neutralizing activity.[138] Using herpesvirus for foreign glycoprotein delivery might prove challenging in some instances, because they encode multiple glycoproteins of their own[137] that might compete for B cell responses, and achieving expression levels needed to elicit immune responses may require specific genetic manipulations.[139]

Cytomegalovirus

Cytomegaloviruses persist indefinitely in their host following primary infection.[140] CMV persistence and the resulting low-level constitutive immune stimulation maintains an expanded pool of effector-differentiated T cells which control infection and prevents CMV disease.[141] This persistent infection held in check by host immunity parallels what occurs in macaques infected with live attenuated SIV. This similarity has prompted the hypothesis that vaccine delivery with replication-competent CMV vectors could generate protective immunity from SIV or HIV infection.[36]

A replication-competent rhesus (Rh) CMV 68-1 vector,[142–144] which has been used as the basis for a multivalent vaccine delivering nearly a complete SIVmac239 proteome, has been studied extensively in the SIVmac239 challenge-protection model.[48,49] In two independent studies conducted in male Indian rhesus macaques, the live vaccine was able to safely establish a persistent infection in animals that were already seropositive for RhCMV and elicit T cell responses against the encoded SIV immunogens. The immunized animals were also able to maintain pools of T cells responsive to an expanded breadth of SIV epitopes.[48,49] Fifty percent of the immunized animals, after intra-rectal SIV challenge, demonstrated rapid and durable control of SIV replication with viral load reduced to very low or undetectable levels. A later study among immunized and intra-vaginally challenged female macaques demonstrated the same vaccine efficacy.[145] It is not understood why stringent immune control was limited to 50% of the animals, but host genetic may play a role as well as the activity of SIV-specific CD8 effector T cells at the time of infection.[146,147] Immunoregulatory factors encoded by RhCMV also play a role in determining the spectrum of recognized epitopes.[148,149]

The preclinical RhCMV-SIV data has prompted the start of a clinical vaccine development program (*L. Picker, personal communication*). Since cytomegaloviruses are host restricted,[140] a new vector is under development based on human CMV (HCMV). Developing a new vector is challenging even though HCMV and RhCMV are biologically homologous. The majority of viral proteins encoded by the rhesus and human viruses are related, but their respective genomes are large and express unique polypeptides and microRNAs.[143,150,151] Additionally, HCMV primary infection during pregnancy is linked to birth defects, and the virus also causes serious complications in some immunosuppressed patients undergoing organ transplants[141,152,153]; therefore, development of an attenuated HCMV vector is essential toward minimizing risk. Fortunately, there is prior experience showing that live attenuated HCMV vaccines can be safely tested in the clinic.[153,154] Progress also has been made toward developing an attenuated HCMV vector by using RhCMV as a model. Focusing on genes that are conserved between HCMV and the rhesus virus, gene knockouts have been identified that attenuate RhCMV replication in vivo but still allow the virus to establish a persistent infection.[155] In considering HCMV as a vector it also is important to consider that seroprevalence is relatively high in humans by an early age.[141] However, preclinical studies mentioned above have shown RhCMV can infect seropositive animals and that preexisting immunity does not prevent responses against the foreign SIV immunogens.

Rhadinovirus

Rhesus macaque rhadinovirus (RRV) establishes a persistent infection in lymphocytes[156] and can serve as a valuable tool for the investigating immunity elicited by a persisting virus that infects lymphoid tissues, particularly as this is considered an important contributor to the efficacy of live attenuated SIV.[157] RRV vectors encoding SIV genes, like RhCMV, can infect seropositive macaques making it possible to deliver SIV immunogens in the presence preexisting immunity. NHPs vaccinated with RRV vectors encoding SIV Gag, Env, and Rev-Tat-Nef antigens had robust and persistent T cell responses, though with an epitope specificity that differed from that elicited by RhCMV-SIV vaccination.[51] Pathogenic SIVmac239 challenge of vaccinated animals resulted in 100% infection; however, chronic viremia was reduced by an average of $1.5-2 \log_{10}$ units. These results, which were lower in magnitude than the viral load reduction seen in macaques vaccinated with RhCMV-SIV, come with the caveat that SIV challenge was administered via intravenous injection rather than the more common method of repeated intrarectal exposure. Despite an ability to induce robust T cell responses, the RRV-SIV Env vector failed to elicit high antibody titers,[51] as was the case with the Env component of the multivalent RhCMV-SIV vaccine.[48] A new Env gene designed with RRV-specific codon usage and controlled with an RRV rather than HCMV promoter has been developed for the RRV vector.[139,158,159] Together, the new promoter and RRV-specific codon optimization has placed the Env gene under control of an RRV-encoded transactivator that modulates the timing of expression during the viral lytic cycle, thereby significantly enhancing Env expression and consequently immunogenicity as measured by higher rates of Env seroconversion in vaccinated macaques.[139]

Varicella Zoster Virus

Varicella zoster virus (VZV), for which there are two licensed live vaccines, establishes a life-long infection that stimulates T cells,[160–162] thus making it a potentially relevant for development of a persisting HIV vaccine delivery vector.[163,164] Despite its potential, VZV is difficult to evaluate preclinically as it is host restricted failing to cause disease in animals other than humans.[165] In NHPs, wild-type virus elicits T cell and antibodies, but infection is aborted before establishing chronic, latent infection.[52,166] As expected, VZV-SIV Env vaccines have been shown to be weakly immunogenic in NHPs.[167] In macaques vaccinated with VZV-SIV, increased SIVsmE660 replication was observed following challenge and was associated with elevated CD4 T cell activation. The study investigators noted that the suboptimal immune responses elicited by host-restricted and attenuated VZV-SIV Env vectors may have established conditions that augmented CD4 T cell activation once SIV infection occurred. In contrast, a simian varicella vector encoding SIV Gag and Env did not cause infection enhancement,[168] suggesting that vector replicative capacity plays an important role in determining the nature of the immune response.

RNA VIRUS VECTORS

A wide variety of RNA viruses have been developed as vectors, partly because there are a number of live attenuated vaccines for RNA viruses already in use, including polio, measles, mumps, and yellow fever (Table 2.1).[169] RNA viruses also are considerably smaller and encode substantially fewer potential vector immunogens than the DNA viruses described above.

POSITIVE-STRAND RNA VIRUSES

Poliovirus was one of the earliest positive-strand RNA viruses to be investigated as an autonomously replicating HIV vaccine vector.[60] The rigid capsid structure of poliovirus and other positive-strand RNA viruses limit their ability to accommodate additional gene inserts. This is one reason why, historically, much of the vector research on this class of viruses has focused on using their genomes to generate self-amplifying RNA replicons rather than replication competent viruses.[33,170–172] The addition of foreign coding sequences can also be complex in positive-strand RNA viruses, as they need to be integrated in a way that does not interfere with specialized mechanisms of protein expression and co-translational or posttranslational processing during the RNA virus life cycle.[173–175]

Yellow Fever Virus

Strain yellow fever virus (YFV) 17D is an attractive vector development candidate, as vaccination with the live attenuated version of the virus has been used for decades to control disease in endemic areas.[176] There have been three principal methods (Fig. 2.2) of inserting foreign sequences into a replication-competent YFV vector.[177] In one, a YFV polypeptide is modified without significant loss of function to carry a relatively small foreign epitope insert. In the second, larger foreign protein sequences were grafted into the

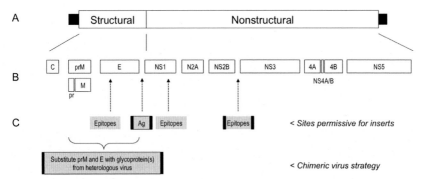

FIGURE 2.2 Strategies used for incorporating foreign sequences into recombinant YFV. The single-stranded, positive-sense RNA genome is shown in Panel A. The coding region for the large precursor polyprotein is divided into regions encoding the structural and nonstructural polypeptides. Co-translational or posttranslational cleavage of the precursor produces polypeptides that are shown in Panel B. Panel C illustrates how foreign amino acid sequences are added to YFV vectors.[175,177,178] Relatively short epitopes have been grafted into permissive sites in the E glycoprotein or NS1. Epitopes flanked by cleavage signals (black) also have been added between NS2B and NS3. Larger antigens derived from SIV or HIV Gag flanked by cleavage signals have been introduced in the region between E and NS1. Finally, the prM and E glycoproteins can be substituted with analogous glycoproteins from other flaviviruses to make chimeras.

YFV polyprotein precursor along with flanking elements to enable correct processing of viral polypeptides as well as the foreign immunogen. In the third approach, chimeric viruses were generated, where the YFV attachment protein was replaced with a foreign functional viral glycoprotein. These strategies have been increasingly successful, particularly for HIV and SIV gene inserts, despite the challenge of maintaining viral fitness through the introduction a foreign sequence that offers no selective advantage.[66,179,180] The positive results have primarily been seen in YFV vectors eliciting potent CD8 T cell responses in rhesus macaques.[66,67,181–183]

Rubella Virus

Rubella virus is another example where there is a long history of safe and effective vaccination with a live-attenuated vaccine indicating that it may hold promise as an efficient and potent vector. It has been engineered to express HIV Gag and Env epitopes, particularly the from the membrane-proximal external region (MPER) of the HIV Env glycoprotein.[62,184,185] The Rubella virus HIV vectors have been shown to elicit high antibody titers and T cell responses in vaccinated rhesus macaques. The vectors also boosted antigen-specific responses even in animals that had seroconverted to rubella virus.[184,186]

Semliki Forest Virus

Semliki forest virus (SFV) RNA replicons have been developed to propagate in membrane vesicles. In the context of an SIV vaccine model, the replicon was constructed to encode the SFV replicase machinery, an SIV immunogen, and the vesicular stomatitis virus (VSV) glycoprotein (G) that enables vesicle budding and propagation.[63,187] Propagating vesicles encoding SIV Gag or Env have been used to safely vaccinate macaques, and when used in a heterologous prime-boost regimen in combination with replicating VSV vectors, animals vaccinated with Gag plus Env developed immunity that protected them from infection following a high-dose intrarectal challenge with SIVsmE660.[64,188,189]

Rhinovirus

Human rhinovirus has been modified to deliver epitopes derived from the HIV Env MPER that are grafted into the viral capsid protein where they are displayed on the surface of the naked virus particle.[190] A study published recently showed that genetically modified mice intranasally infected with the human rhinovirus vector vaccine generated antibodies against MPER sequences.[191] Recently, an alternative strategy for inserting larger sequences has been developed in which the foreign polypeptide is flanked by polyprotein processing signals,[192] resembling the approach used for inserting sequences in the YFV polyprotein (Fig. 2.2).

DOUBLE-STRANDED RNA VIRUSES (REOVIRUS)

The Reoviridae family may provide the foundation for vectors that can deliver vaccine immunogens to the gastrointestinal tract where they can stimulate local immunity at the rectal mucosal barrier and underlying tissues. Rotavirus, the prototypical member of this virus family, and the licensed vaccines developed against it, demonstrate that reoviruses can elicit effective mucosal immunity.[193] However, the introduction of foreign sequences into a reovirus vector is complicated for several reasons: (1) they have segmented double-stranded RNA genomes[194]; (2) gene segment packaging signals overlap with coding sequences[68]; and (3) the icosahedral capsid limits gene insert capacity.[194] Reverse genetic systems may overcome some of these obstacles,[195] given that successful strategies have been developed for adding foreign sequences into 3 of 10 orthoreovirus gene segments.[68] In one system a reovirus vector encoding 300 amino acids from SIV Gag was shown to elicit Gag-specific T cells in mice,[68] but further research is required to determine if a reovirus vector can be used for gastrointestinal delivery of an HIV immunogen and whether this can be extended for use in humans where preexisting immunity to reoviruses is common.[196]

NEGATIVE-STRAND RNA VIRUSES

As a group, the enveloped RNA viruses with single-stranded negative sense genomes have been one of the more intensively investigated as vector candidates.[37,197,198] Among the reasons are their use as live attenuated vaccines in both humans and animals (Table 2.1), including vaccines against measles, mumps, canine distemper, rinderpest, bovine parainfluenza, and Newcastle disease.[12,13,199–201] As most of these viruses infect by the oral or respiratory route, they may be well suited for mucosal administration. Despite some challenges in manipulating genomes of single-stranded negative-sense RNA viruses,[202,203] these pathogens also offer the advantage of having no rigid capsid structure and being refractory to homologous recombination.[37,197,202,204]

Vesicular Stomatitis Virus

VSV recently has been used as a vector platform for a promising Ebola virus vaccine candidate (see below), but was actually one of the earliest RNA viruses developed for use as a live vaccine vector in the field of HIV vaccinology.[37] Rose and colleagues generated prototype vectors for delivery of SIV Gag and HIV Env that were found to be safe when administered to rhesus macaques by multiple routes.[84] Vaccinated animals were able to achieve viremic control when challenged with SHIV infection. Some of the success may have been on account of the innovative design in which the second and third vaccine doses were with vectors in which the G protein from different VSV serotypes were used to minimize the interference of anti-vector immunity.[84,85] A Phase I clinical trial followed the NHP studies with a VSV vector (VSV-N4CT1-Gag1) that was modified to decrease viral propagation and neuroviru-lence potential.[205,206] The highest intramuscular dose of this vaccine demon-strated safety and Gag-specific T cell responses in approximately 60% of volunteers.[207] A second Phase I trial with a plasmid DNA vaccine prime and a VSV-N4CT1-Gag1 vector boost showing promising immunogenicity results as well.[208,209] An Env (clade C.1086) vaccine candidate based on this attenuated VSV platform also is being advanced to clinical trials (*David Clarke and John Eldridge, personal communication*). Additional VSV-HIV vaccine constructs have been developed and tested in NHP models[64,208,210–212], and despite their greater capacity for replication compared to the vector evaluated in humans, adverse reactions have not been noted. Various replication-competent VSV vector designs have been evaluated that express different forms of Env or Env epitopes[213–216] including chimeric viruses the encode functional Env (see below). Overall, replication-competent VSV vector vaccines have been shown to be immunogenic, especially when administered via the mucosal route and as part of a heterologous prime-boost regimen.

Rabies Virus

Live vectors based on rabies virus (RV)[79,80] have been developed using a G serotype exchange strategy similar to those developed for VSV.[84,85] In SIV or SHIV models of rhesus macaque infection, RV vector vaccination has evoked both T and B cell responses[79,80] and reduced SIVmac251 viremia[79] or pro-vided protection from SHIV89.6 disease.[80] Murine studies also have shown that RV-HIV Gag vaccines can be combined with other vectors in heterolo-gous prime-boost regimens to achieve an increased magnitude of T cell response.[217] These vectors also have been modified so as reduce RV's risk of neurovirulence.[218] One of the more innovative modifications to RV vectors is based on the finding that mutant RV lacking the matrix gene (ΔM) propagates less efficiently, however gene expression remains relatively unaffected.[219] Recently, a ΔM vector encoding Env was shown to elicit anti-SIV Env antibo-dies in vaccinated mice with or without a heterologous boost, suggesting that this technology might be useful in development of HIV Env delivery vaccines.[220]

Sendai Virus

Sendai virus (SeV) naturally infects the respiratory tract of rodents,[221] thus it has been targeted for development of replication-competent intranasal vac-cine delivery vectors.[222] A live SeV-SIV Gag vector was evaluated in maca-ques and found to be safe and immunogenic when delivered by the intranasal route. Animals vaccinated with a regimen of DNA prime followed by intranasal boost were able to exert substantial control over SIVmac239 replication following IV challenge compared to control animals infected with the highly pathogenic virus.[81] Based on this positive preclinical finding, a vector encoding HIV Gag was advanced for clinical evaluation of the first intranasal HIV vaccine (ClinicalTrials.gov Identifier: NCT01705990). The SeV-Gag phase 1 trial was designed to evaluate immunogenicity following intranasal vaccination, assess SeV and Ad35 in a heterologous prime-boost regimen, and also monitor the potential effects of preexisting cross-reacting human parainfluenza virus type 1 antibodies,[223] which preclinical studies predicted would not interfere with intranasal vaccination.[224] The phase I study results showed that the vaccine was safe and effectively primed Gag-specific cellular immune responses, as the combination of intranasal SeV-Gag prime and intramuscular Ad35-GRIN (GRIN: Gag-Reverse transcriptase-integrase-Nef; [225]) elicited Gag specific T cells in a high percentage (~90%) of clinical trial volunteers.[226] SeV vectors capable of expressing HIV Env spikes are being advanced for evaluation in macaques (*C. Parks and T. Matano, unpublished*).

Newcastle Disease Virus

Newcastle disease virus (NDV) is a paramyxovirus that infects large poultry populations and is controlled by mass vaccination using a modified live vaccine.[201] Attenuated NDV strains are being investigated as both vaccine delivery vectors and oncolytic agents.[227–229] A number of human clinical trials have been conducted safely with the oncolytic viruses.[230,231] Initially, NDV vectors were developed as vehicles for the delivery of SIV or HIV Gag. Murine studies demonstrated that intranasal vaccination with these vectors was safe and elicited Gag-specific T cell response.[76,217,232] Progress also has been made in the construction of NDV vectors that deliver HIV Env immunogens. Specifically, NDV vectors encoding gp160, gp140 or gp120 have been shown to be immunogenic in small animals vaccinated mucosally or by intramuscular injection.[77,233] Notably, vectors encoding gp160 incorporate Env in the virus particle, suggesting that NDV might be a promising platform for Env spike delivery.[77] In fact, novel vectors have been developed that direct budding of Gag-Env particles from infected cells.[234] Moreover, co-delivery of Env plus Gag has been shown to enhance immunogenicity in murine models.[234,235]

Mumps Virus and Parainfluenza Virus Type 5

Two rubulaviruses—one Mumps virus (MuV) used as a live attenuated vaccine to prevent Mumps disease in humans,[12,236] and the other parainfluenza virus type 5 (PIV5) that causes "kennel cough" in dogs[237]—are the basis for two HIV vector vaccines. The MuV-HIV vector expresses HIV Gag and has been safely tested in macaques. In a heterologous prime-boost regimen that included this vector and the attenuated VSV-N4CT1-Gag1 vaccine described earlier, strong T cell responses were induced when the MuV-Gag vector was used as the prime.[75] The immunogenicity of a PIV5 vector encoding HIV Env gp160 was also assessed in African green monkeys.[83] Mucosal vaccination via the intranasal and intratracheal routes elicited Env binding antibodies. Notably, detectable Env antibodies were elicited without using a heterologous boost, suggesting that the PIV5 vector might have potential applications as a delivery platform for the HIV Env trimer.[83]

Measles Virus and Canine Distemper Virus

Measles virus (MeV) and canine distemper virus (CDV) are related morbilliviruses.[238] Immunization with modified live vaccines[199,239,240] controls both of these highly infectious pathogens. Since they are naturally lymphotropic,[241,242] the morbilliviruses provide a vector platform that can be used to mimic a prominent feature of attenuated SIVmac239 strains that elicit protective immunity.[157,243,244] Furthermore, the availability of safe, live morbillivirus vaccine strains offers an advantage for the development and testing of prototype vectors; and recent results indicate that the attenuated viruses may replicate in antigen-presenting dendritic cells.[245] Cells infected with morbilliviruses might also persist following infection,[246] which may help to evoke durable immune responses. When administered parentally like the live measles-mumps-rubella vaccine, MeV-HIV vectors have been shown to be safe and immunogenic in rhesus macaques.[72,73,247]

Preexisting immunity generated by widespread measles vaccination is a potential limitation for the use of MeV vectors. Although the modest serum antibody titers induced by measles vaccination are significantly lower than those generated by natural infection,[248,249] they still may reduce the potency of a MeV vector. Strategies to minimize interference from preexisting antibodies include mucosal vaccine administration,[224,250,251] higher dose vaccination, or substitution of glycoproteins from CDV[252] or other more distantly related viruses.[253,254] CDV is being investigated as a vector, not only as an alternative to MeV, but also to take advantage of how it targets the lymphoid tissue during infection and the low prevalence of preexisting immunity.[69,252,255] In considering a potential path to clinical development for a CDV vector, it is important to note that no human diseases are associated with the canine virus[256] and that attenuated CDV[257] was previously tested safely in humans.[258,259] Evaluation of both CDV-SIV and CDV-HIV vectors is ongoing in macaques, and preliminary results indicate that they have been safe and immunogenic thus far (*J. Zhang, G. Morrow, and C. Parks, unpublished*).

Influenza Virus

The use of a licensed, live-attenuated influenza vaccine (FluMist®) makes replicating influenza virus a potential candidate as a mucosal vector, particularly as the intranasal vaccine has been shown to provide more durable cross-reactive immunity in some age groups compared to the traditional inactivated subviral vaccines.[260,261] The segmented genome of influenza virus differentiates it from virus vectors described above. However, technology used to generate recombinant influenza virus shares some features with methods used for viruses with nonsegmented genomes.[203] Nonetheless, the development of genetically stable vectors can be more challenging for influenza, as the eight influenza virus gene segments have a more restricted capacity for foreign sequence insertion, gene segment packaging signals overlap with viral polypeptide coding sequences, and the gene segments can reassort if coinfection occurs.[262,263] Still, influenza vectors have advanced to preclinical testing in small animal and nonhuman primate models. Recently, influenza virus vectors containing HIV Env MPER epitopes were grafted into the influenza hemagglutinin (HA) glycoprotein[70] without a decrement in HA function needed for virus propagation. Guinea pigs vaccinated with the recombinant influenza virus developed MPER-specific antibodies, though HIV pseudovirus neutralization activity was low. Similar results were obtained with MPER grafts into VSV G protein,[214] indicating that MPER immunogenicity will need to be augmented to elicit substantial B-cell responses when the short epitope is displayed as a graft within a heterologous glycoprotein.

Foreign epitopes fused to the HA or neuraminidase (NA) glycoproteins might prove to be better T cell inducers through intranasal vaccination with live influenza virus vectors. Sequence motifs from HIV Gag, Env, and Tat grafted onto HA elicited T cell responses[264,265] in mice. Similarly, elements from SIV Gag and Tat incorporated in influenza virus NA induced T cell responses in pigtail macaques that were vaccinated intranasally.[71,266] In the macaque studies, SIV challenge resulted in SIVmac239 mutations that were consistent with immune pressure resulting from live influenza virus vector vaccination. As these authors noted, the induction of SIV-specific immune responses by the intranasal influenza virus vector was encouraging, but broader epitope coverage would be necessary to elicit protective immunity, which is consistent with results seen with live YFV vaccines delivering limited numbers of SIV T cell epitopes.[181]

ENVELOPED RNA VIRUS CHIMERAS

Recombinant enveloped RNA viruses that can be modified to use functional heterologous viral glycoproteins as their attachment proteins provide a unique vector platform for delivering viral transmembrane glycoprotein immunogens. Their dependence on expression of the foreign viral glycoprotein for virus propagation provides strong selective pressure to ensure that at least some of the expressed immunogen is functionally configured and arrayed on the virus particle. The live chimeric virus strategy is proving to be very successful for other vaccines, including the YFV/Japanese encephalitis virus chimera[267] licensed for use in some countries under the name Imojev® (Fig. 2.2).[30] Also, the candidate Ebola virus vaccine based on a live VSV-Ebola chimera[268] was rapidly advanced to clinical trial and found to be highly efficacious when used in a ring vaccination trial.[269−272]

In the context of HIV, the chimeric virus design has distinct advantages for delivery of trimeric Env spikes, but it can be challenging to implement as a live Env vaccine for a number of reasons. For example, replacement of the native viral glycoprotein with Env tends to attenuate replication. Additionally, Env modifications have been required to generate genetically stable vectors that express Env and propagate efficiently.[65,74,273] Furthermore, the modified cell tropism determined by Env affects the biology of the virus, thus safety and immunogenicity must be determined empirically in an NHP model that will support replication of a CD4/CCR5-dependent chimeric virus. The importance of evaluation of chimeric viruses in an animal model is well illustrated by a variety VSV chimeras in which replacement of VSV G with glycoproteins from Ebola virus, Marburg virus, Lassa fever virus, or lymphocytic choriomeningitis virus was found to substantially reduce the neurovirulence potential associated with unmodified VSV strains.[274−276]

Venezuelan Equine Encephalitis Virus (VEEV)-SHIV, VSV-HIV, and MeV-HIV Chimeras

VEEV is an alphavirus, and accordingly, it is an enveloped virus that has a single-stranded, positive-sense RNA genome. A replication-competent chimera was generated that uses HIV Env as it attachment protein and a novel modified SIV Gag to package the genomic RNA.[65] A study in macaques showed that the CD4/CCR5-dependent VEEV-SHIV chimera was safe and elicited Env antibodies capable of neutralizing tier-1 SIV pseudoviruses without requiring a heterologous boost (*R. Johnston, K. Young, V. Traina-Dorge, J. Whitley, C. LaBranche, D. Montefiori, and C. Jurgens, personal communication*), which may be due in part to VEEV RNA replication triggering intracellular antiviral responses with adjuvanting properties.[277,278]

Enveloped, negative-strand RNA viruses also have been used to generate HIV Env-dependent chimeric viruses. Building on earlier findings that showed VSV particles could be pseudotyped with Env,[279,280] Rose and colleagues generated a replication-competent chimeric VSV that expressed HIV Env in place of VSV G (Fig. 2.3) and was dependent on cellular HIV

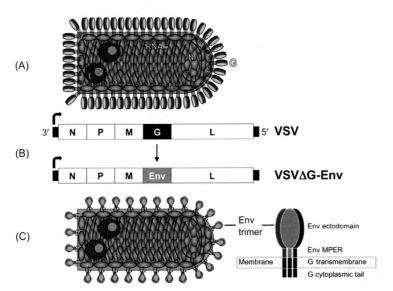

FIGURE 2.3 VSVΔG-Env chimeric virus vaccine. The figure illustrates the design of a VSVΔG-Env chimera. (A) Schematic of the VSV particle, which is composed of 5 viral structural proteins[286]: *N*, nucleocapsid; *P*, phosphoprotein; *M*: matrix protein; *G*, glycoprotein; and *L*, large protein. The *L* and *P* proteins are subunits of the RNA-dependent RNA polymerase, which is present in the virus particle. (B) The linear map of the single-stranded, negative-sense, nonsegmented RNA genome of VSV is shown at the top. The HIV Env-dependent VSVΔG-Env chimeric virus genome is shown below the VSV map. (C) Schematic showing that the VSVΔG-Env contains Env spikes on the surface of the virus particle. In the chimeric virus described in the text, the transmembrane region and cytoplasmic tail[281] is replaced with analogous sequences from VSV G. The hybrid protein retains functions needed for direct infection of CD4+ / CCR5+ cells.

coreceptors for productive infection.[273] A replication-competent MeV-SIV chimera encoding SIV Env in place of the MeV F and H glycoproteins also has been developed using the attenuated Schwarz vaccine strain of MeV.[74] A live VSV-HIV Env chimera encoding modified clade A HIV Env in place of VSV G (Fig. 2.3, ΔG) has been advanced for evaluation in the macaque model (*G. Morrow, M. Yuan, W. Koff, C. Parks, unpublished*). Administration of the live chimera to nasopharyngeal mucosal surfaces of NHPs caused no observable adverse reactions and the animals developed Env-specific antibodies. The vaccinated macaques also were found to be protected from repeated rectal challenge with SHIV SF162 p3 compared to placebo controls. This VSV-Env chimeric virus vaccine and the immune responses it elicited will be studied further, but early results indicate that neutralizing serum antibodies were not responsible for resistance to SHIV infection. Planning for continued preclinical evaluation and development of a clinical trial candidate is in progress.

CONCLUSIONS

As recently as a decade ago, relatively few replication-competent viral vectors were being developed and rigorously evaluated as vaccine candidates.[26] Multiple challenges hindered the advancement of this vaccine platform in the past, including: (1) concerns about the safety of replicating viral vectors, particularly among immunocompromised individuals; (2) difficulties in balancing the replicative capacity of a viral vector with the appropriate level of attenuation to ensure both immunogenicity and safety; (3) technical hurdles to modifying viruses so that they are both genetically stable and propagate to high titers; (4) the costs and capabilities needed for testing candidate vaccines in multiple animal models. Nevertheless, as illustrated by the examples described above, significant progress has been made in the development of a variety of vectors with varying biological properties some of which may be best suited to eliciting T cell responses (i.e., CMV, replicating adenovirus vectors) while others have been designed primarily to deliver spike glycoprotein immunogens (i.e., chimeric viruses).

In the context of HIV there is a strong possibility that vectors could be used to mimic key properties of the efficacious SIVmac239Δnef vaccine. Individually, many of the vectors briefly reviewed share some features with this experimental live SIV vaccine. Thus, as rigorous vaccine vector candidate assessments are carried out in NHP challenge-protection models, and in some cases human clinical trials, valuable data will be produced that might help identify those vector platform characteristics that can make a meaningful contribution to vaccine effectiveness. The ability to replicate and produce virus progeny that initiates subsequent rounds of infection and provide sustained antigen expression is a key feature of live vectors, but also their ability to evade various pathogen recognition pathways and cellular antiviral responses will provide distinctive immunostimulatory properties to RNA[282,283] or DNA[36,130,284,285] virus vectors. Their unique abilities to trigger and regulate the antiviral response in vivo will make it informative to include gene expression profiling in preclinical and clinical studies to understand how the innate antiviral response might be contributing to vaccine immunogenicity and efficacy. Similarly, cell tropism will have a significant effect on innate and adaptive immune responses, and several vectors reviewed above, such as measles and CDVs, target lymphoid cells, which may be an important tropism for the generation of potent and durable immune responses against SIV or HIV.

Finally, many of the newer vectors are being designed so they are not inhibited by preexisting immunity and are more efficient at stimulating immunity at mucosal barriers. One way of achieving the former is to use viruses that either have infrequent contact with humans (i.e., NDV, VSV, simian Ad) or human viruses where seroprevalence is low (alternative Ad serotypes). The chimeric virus approach also replaces the main target of anti-vector antibodies with antigen of interest. Vectors being developed that can be administered to mucosal surfaces might also lessen some effects of preexisting immunity. Rigorous evaluation of these vectors in animal models and eventual humans will ultimately determine their benefits for vaccine development and the mitigation of human disease.

ACKNOWLEDGMENTS

The author thanks Lisa Gieber and Sandi Glass for their assistance with manuscript research and composition, Gavin Morrow and Jason Zhang for helpful reviews, and multiple colleagues for making unpublished research available, including Drs. Louis Picker (Oregon Health and Science University), Giuseppe Pantaleo (Swiss Vaccine Research Institute), Robert Johnston (Global Vaccines, Inc.), John Eldridge (Profectus Biosciences, Inc.), Tetsuro Matano (National Institute of Infectious Diseases, AIDS Research Center, Japan), and Ron Desrosiers (University of Miami). IAVI's work is made possible by generous support from many donors including: the Bill & Melinda Gates Foundation; the Ministry of Foreign Affairs of Denmark; Irish Aid; the Ministry of Finance of Japan; the Ministry of Foreign Affairs of the Netherlands; the Norwegian Agency for Development Cooperation (NORAD); the United Kingdom Department for International Development (DFID), and the United States Agency for International Development (USAID). The full list of IAVI donors is available at www.iavi.org. The contents are the responsibility of the International AIDS Vaccine Initiative and do not necessarily reflect the views of USAID or the United States Government.

REFERENCES

1. O'Connell RJ, Kim JH, Corey L, Michael NL. Human immunodeficiency virus vaccine trials. *Cold Spring Harb Perspect Med* 2012;**2**(12):a007351.
2. Girard MP, Koff WC. Human immunodeficiency virus vaccines. In: Plotkin SA, Orenstein WA, Offit PA, editors. *Vaccines*. 6th ed. Philadelphia: Elsevier Saunders; 2013. p. 1097−121.
3. Kim JH, Excler JL, Michael NL. Lessons from the RV144 Thai phase III HIV-1 vaccine trial and the search for correlates of protection. *Annu Rev Med* 2015;**66**:423−37.
4. Tomaras GD, Haynes BF. Advancing toward HIV-1 vaccine efficacy through the intersections of immune correlates. *Vaccines (Basel)* 2014;**2**(1):15−35.
5. Rerks-Ngarm S, Pitisuttithum P, Nitayaphan S, Kaewkungwal J, Chiu J, Paris R, et al. Vaccination with ALVAC and AIDSVAX to prevent HIV-1 infection in Thailand. *N Eng J Med* 2009;**361**(23):2209−20.
6. Corey L, Gilbert PB, Tomaras GD, Haynes BF, Pantaleo G, Fauci AS. Immune correlates of vaccine protection against HIV-1 acquisition. *Sci Transl Med* 2015;**7**(310). 310rv7.
7. Buchbinder SP, Mehrotra DV, Duerr A, Fitzgerald DW, Mogg R, Li D, et al. Efficacy assessment of a cell-mediated immunity HIV-1 vaccine (the Step Study): a double-blind, randomised, placebo-controlled, test-of-concept trial. *Lancet* 2008;**372**(9653):1881−93.
8. McElrath MJ, De Rosa SC, Moodie Z, Dubey S, Kierstead L, Janes H, et al. HIV-1 vaccine-induced immunity in the test-of-concept step study: a case-cohort analysis. *Lancet* 2008;**372** (9653):1894−905.

9. Gray GE, Allen M, Moodie Z, Churchyard G, Bekker LG, Nchabeleng M, et al. Safety and efficacy of the HVTN 503/Phambili study of a clade-B-based HIV-1 vaccine in South Africa: a double-blind, randomised, placebo-controlled test-of-concept phase 2b study. *Lancet Infect Dis* 2011;**11**(7):507−15.

10. Berk AJ. Adenoviridae: the viruses and their replication. In: Fields BN, Knipe DM, Howley PM, Griffin DE, Lamb RA, Martin MA, editors. *Fields virology*, vol. 2. New York: Lippincott, Williams, and Wilkins; 2007. p. 2371−3.

11. Appaiahgari MB, Vrati S. Adenoviruses as gene/vaccine delivery vectors: promises and pitfalls. *Expert Opin Biol Ther* 2015;**15**(3):337−51.

12. Minor PD. Live attenuated vaccines: historical successes and current challenges. *Virology* 2015;**479-480**:379−92.

13. Plotkin SL, Plotkin SA. A short history of vaccination. In: Plotkin SA, Orenstein WA, Offit PA, editors. *Vaccines*. 6th ed. Philadelphia: Elsevier Saunders; 2013. p. 1−13.

14. Meeusen EN, Walker J, Peters A, Pastoret PP, Jungersen G. Current status of veterinary vaccines. *Clin Microbiol Rev* 2007;**20**(3):489−510.

15. Daniel MD, Kirchhoff F, Czajak SC, Sehgal PK, Desrosiers RC. Protective effects of a live attenuated SIV vaccine with a deletion in the nef gene. *Science* 1992;**258**(5090):1938−41.

16. Koff WC, Johnson PR, Watkins DI, Burton DR, Lifson JD, Hasenkrug KJ, et al. HIV vaccine design: insights from live attenuated SIV vaccines. *Nat Immunol* 2006;**7**(1):19−23.

17. Jia B, Ng SK, DeGottardi MQ, Piatak M, Yuste E, Carville A, et al. Immunization with single-cycle SIV significantly reduces viral loads after an intravenous challenge with SIV (mac)239. *PLoS Pathog* 2009;**5**(1):e1000272.

18. Johnson RP, Lifson JD, Czajak SC, Cole KS, Manson KH, Glickman R, et al. Highly attenuated vaccine strains of simian immunodeficiency virus protect against vaginal challenge: inverse relationship of degree of protection with level of attenuation. *J Virol* 1999;**73**(6):4952−61.

19. Johnson RP, Desrosiers RC. Protective immunity induced by live attenuated simian immunodeficiency virus. *Curr Opin Immunol* 1998;**10**(4):436−43.

20. Reynolds MR, Weiler AM, Piaskowski SM, Piatak Jr. M, Robertson HT, Allison DB, et al. A trivalent recombinant Ad5 gag/pol/nef vaccine fails to protect rhesus macaques from infection or control virus replication after a limiting-dose heterologous SIV challenge. *Vaccine* 2012;**30**(30):4465−75.

21. Plotkin SA, Orenstein WA, Offit PA. *Vaccines*. 6th ed. Philadelphia: Elsevier Saunders; 2013.

22. Vaccines, Blood & Biologics-Approved Products [Internet]. U.S. Department of Health and Human Services. Available from: http://www.fda.gov/BiologicsBloodVaccines/Vaccines/ApprovedProducts/default.htm; 2016 [cited January 2016].

23. Behbehani AM. The smallpox story: life and death of an old disease. *Microbiol Rev* 1983;**47**(4):455−509.

24. Sutter RW, Kew OM, Cochi SL, Aylward BR. Poliovirus vaccine-live. In: Plotkin SA, Orenstein WA, Offit PA, editors. *Vaccines*. 6th ed. Philadelphia: Elsevier Saunders; 2013. p. 598−645.

25. Whitney JB, Ruprecht RM. Live attenuated HIV vaccines: pitfalls and prospects. *Curr Opin Infect Dis* 2004;**17**(1):17−26.

26. Koff WC, Parks CL, Berkhout B, Ackland J, Noble S, Gust ID. Replicating viral vectors as HIV vaccines Summary Report from IAVI Sponsored Satellite Symposium, International AIDS Society Conference, July 22, 2007. *Biologicals* 2008;**36**(5):277−86.

27. Hitt MM, Graham FL. Adenovirus vectors for human gene therapy. *Adv Virus Res* 2000;**55**:479−505.

28. Danthinne X, Imperiale MJ. Production of first generation adenovirus vectors: a review. *Gene Ther* 2000;**7**(20):1707−14.

29. Draper SJ, Heeney JL. Viruses as vaccine vectors for infectious diseases and cancer. *Nat Rev Microbiol* 2010;**8**(1):62−73.

30. Guy B, Guirakhoo F, Barban V, Higgs S, Monath TP, Lang J. Preclinical and clinical development of YFV 17D-based chimeric vaccines against dengue, West Nile and Japanese encephalitis viruses. *Vaccine* 2010;**28**(3):632−49.

31. Robert-Guroff M. Replicating and nonreplicating viral vectors for vaccine development. *Curr Opin Biotechnol* 2007;**18**(6):546−56.

32. Patterson LJ, Robert-Guroff M. Replicating adenovirus vector prime/protein boost strategies for HIV vaccine development. *Expert Opin Biol Ther* 2008;**8**(9):1347−63.

33. Liniger M, Zuniga A, Naim HY. Use of viral vectors for the development of vaccines. *Expert Rev Vaccines* 2007;**6**(2):255 66.

34. Li S, Locke E, Bruder J, Clarke D, Doolan DL, Havenga MJ, et al. Viral vectors for malaria vaccine development. *Vaccine* 2007;**25**(14):2567−74.

35. Excler JL, Parks CL, Ackland J, Rees H, Gust ID, Koff WC. Replicating viral vectors as HIV vaccines: summary report from the IAVI-sponsored satellite symposium at the AIDS vaccine 2009 conference. *Biologicals* 2010;**38**(4):511−21.

36. Picker LJ, Hansen SG, Lifson JD. New paradigms for HIV/AIDS vaccine development. *Annu Rev Med* 2012;**63**:95−111.

37. Clarke DK, Cooper D, Egan MA, Hendry RM, Parks CL, Udem SA. Recombinant vesicular stomatitis virus as an HIV-1 vaccine vector. *Springer Semin Immunopathol* 2006;**28**(3):239−53.

38. Parks CL, Picker LJ, King CR. Development of replication-competent viral vectors for HIV vaccine delivery. *Curr Opin HIV AIDS* 2013;**8**(5):402−11.

39. Deng S, Martin C, Patil R, Zhu F, Zhao B, Xiang Z, et al. Vaxvec: The first web-based recombinant vaccine vector database and its data analysis. *Vaccine* 2015;**33**(48):6938−46.

40. Alexander J, Mendy J, Vang L, Avanzini JB, Garduno F, Manayani DJ, et al. Pre-clinical development of a recombinant, replication-competent adenovirus serotype 4 vector vaccine expressing HIV-1 envelope 1086 clade C. *PLoS One* 2013;**8**(12):e82380.

41. Gurwith M, Lock M, Taylor EM, Ishioka G, Alexander J, Mayall T, et al. Safety and immunogenicity of an oral, replicating adenovirus serotype 4 vector vaccine for H5N1 influenza: a randomised, double-blind, placebo-controlled, phase 1 study. *Lancet Infect Dis* 2013;**13**(3):238−50.

42. Patterson LJ, Kuate S, Daltabuit-Test M, Li Q, Xiao P, McKinnon K, et al. Replicating adenovirus-simian immunodeficiency virus (SIV) vectors efficiently prime SIV-specific systemic and mucosal immune responses by targeting myeloid dendritic cells and persisting in rectal macrophages, regardless of immunization route. *Clin Vaccine Immunol* 2012;**19**(5):629−37.

43. Xiao P, Patterson LJ, Kuate S, Brocca-Cofano E, Thomas MA, Venzon D, et al. Replicating adenovirus-simian immunodeficiency virus (SIV) recombinant priming and envelope protein boosting elicits localized, mucosal IgA immunity in rhesus macaques correlated with delayed acquisition following a repeated low-dose rectal SIV(mac251) challenge. *J Virol* 2012;**86**(8):4644−57.

44. Weaver EA, Nehete PN, Buchl SS, Senac JS, Palmer D, Ng P, et al. Comparison of replication-competent, first generation, and helper-dependent adenoviral vaccines. *PLoS One* 2009;**4**(3):e5059.

45. Maxfield LF, Abbink P, Stephenson KE, Borducchi EN, Ng'ang'a D, Kirilova MM, et al. Attenuation of Replication-Competent Adenovirus Serotype 26 Vaccines by Vectorization. *Clin Vaccine Immunol* 2015;**22**(11):1166−75.

46. Abbink P, Maxfield LF, Barouch DH. *Development of replication-competent adenovirus based vaccine vectors. AIDS vaccine 2012.* Boston, Massachusetts, USA: Retrovirology; 2012. p. 310.

47. Handley SA, Thackray LB, Zhao G, Presti R, Miller AD, Droit L, et al. Pathogenic simian immunodeficiency virus infection is associated with expansion of the enteric virome. *Cell* 2012;**151**(2):253−66.

48. Hansen SG, Vieville C, Whizin N, Coyne-Johnson L, Siess DC, Drummond DD, et al. Effector memory T cell responses are associated with protection of rhesus monkeys from mucosal simian immunodeficiency virus challenge. *Nat Med* 2009;**15**(3):293−9.

49. Hansen SG, Ford JC, Lewis MS, Ventura AB, Hughes CM, Coyne-Johnson L, et al. Profound early control of highly pathogenic SIV by an effector memory T-cell vaccine. *Nature* 2011;**473**(7348):523−7.

50. Murphy CG, Lucas WT, Means RE, Czajak S, Hale CL, Lifson JD, et al. Vaccine protection against simian immunodeficiency virus by recombinant strains of herpes simplex virus. *J Virol* 2000;**74**(17):7745−54.

51. Bilello JP, Manrique JM, Shin YC, Lauer W, Li W, Lifson JD, et al. Vaccine protection against simian immunodeficiency virus in monkeys using recombinant gamma-2 herpesvirus. *J Virol* 2011;**85**(23):12708−20.

52. Willer DO, Ambagala AP, Pilon R, Chan JK, Fournier J, Brooks J, et al. Experimental infection of Cynomolgus Macaques (*Macaca fascicularis*) with human varicella-zoster virus. *J Virol* 2012;**86**(7):3626−34.

53. Shao Y, Li T, Wolf H, Liu Y, Liu Y, Wang H, et al. The safety and immunogenicity of HIV-1 vaccines based on DNA and replication-competent vaccina virus vector in phase 1 clinical trial. AIDS Vaccine 2009; October 19, 2009; Retrovirology; Paris, France: 2009. p. 404.

54. Kibler KV, Gomez CE, Perdiguero B, Wong S, Huynh T, Holechek S, et al. Improved NYVAC-based vaccine vectors. *PLoS One* 2011;**6**(11):e25674.

55. Quakkelaar ED, Redeker A, Haddad EK, Harari A, McCaughey SM, Duhen T, et al. Improved innate and adaptive immunostimulation by genetically modified HIV-1 protein expressing NYVAC vectors. *PLoS One* 2011;**6**(2):e16819.

56. Dai K, Liu Y, Liu M, Xu J, Huang W, Huang X, et al. Pathogenicity and immunogenicity of recombinant Tiantan vaccinia virus with deleted C12L and A53R genes. *Vaccine* 2008;**26**(39):5062−71.

57. Zhu R, Huang W, Wang W, Liu Q, Nie J, Meng S, et al. Comparison on virulence and immunogenicity of two recombinant vaccinia vaccines, Tian Tan and Guang9 strains, expressing the HIV-1 envelope gene. *PLoS One* 2012;**7**(11):e48343.

58. Zhang X, Sobue T, Isshiki M, Makino S, Inoue M, Kato K, et al. Elicitation of both anti HIV-1 Env humoral and cellular immunities by replicating vaccinia prime Sendai virus boost regimen and boosting by CD40Lm. *PLoS One* 2012;**7**(12):e51633.

59. Gu R, Stagnar C, Zaichenko L, Ramsingh AI. Induction of mucosal HIV-specific B and T cell responses after oral immunization with live coxsackievirus B4 recombinants. *Vaccine* 2012;**30**(24):3666−74.

60. Crotty S, Miller CJ, Lohman BL, Neagu MR, Compton L, Lu D, et al. Protection against simian immunodeficiency virus vaginal challenge by using Sabin poliovirus vectors. *J Virol* 2001;**75**(16):7435−52.

61. Crotty S, Andino R. Poliovirus vaccine strains as mucosal vaccine vectors and their potential use to develop an AIDS vaccine. *Adv Drug Deliv Rev* 2004;**56**(6):835−52.

62. Virnik K, Ni Y, Berkower I. Live attenuated rubella viral vectors stably express HIV and SIV vaccine antigens while reaching high titers. *Vaccine* 2012;**30**(37):5453−8.

63. Rose NF, Publicover J, Chattopadhyay A, Rose JK. Hybrid alphavirus-rhabdovirus propagating replicon particles are versatile and potent vaccine vectors. *Proc Natl Acad Sci USA* 2008;**105**(15):5839−43.

64. Schell JB, Rose NF, Bahl K, Diller K, Buonocore L, Hunter M, et al. Significant protection against high-dose simian immunodeficiency virus challenge conferred by a new prime-boost vaccine regimen. *J Virol* 2011;**85**(12):5764−72.

65. Jurgens CK, Young KR, Madden VJ, Johnson PR, Johnston RE. A novel self-replicating chimeric lentivirus-like particle. *J Virol* 2012;**86**(1):246−61.

66. Bonaldo MC, Martins MA, Rudersdorf R, Mudd PA, Sacha JB, Piaskowski SM, et al. Recombinant yellow fever vaccine virus 17D expressing simian immunodeficiency virus SIVmac239 gag induces SIV-specific CD8+ T-cell responses in rhesus macaques. *J Virol* 2010;**84**(7):3699−706.

67. Martins MA, Bonaldo MC, Rudersdorf RA, Piaskowski SM, Rakasz EG, Weisgrau KL, et al. Immunogenicity of seven new recombinant yellow fever viruses 17D expressing fragments of SIVmac239 Gag, Nef, and Vif in Indian rhesus macaques. *PLoS One* 2013;**8**(1): e54434.

68. Demidenko AA, Blattman JN, Blattman NN, Greenberg PD, Nibert ML. Engineering recombinant reoviruses with tandem repeats and a tetravirus 2A-like element for exogenous polypeptide expression. *Proc Natl Acad Sci USA* 2013;**110**(20):E1867−76.

69. Zhang X, Richlak S, Nguyen HT, Wallace O, Morrow G, Caulfield M, et al. Development of chimeric HIV Env immunogens for mucosal delivery with attenuated canine distemper virus (CDV) vaccine vectors. *Retrovirology* 2012;**9**(Suppl. 2):P298.

70. Zang Y, Du D, Li N, Su W, Liu X, Zhang Y, et al. Eliciting neutralizing antibodies against the membrane proximal external region of HIV-1 Env by chimeric live attenuated influenza A virus vaccines. *Vaccine* 2015;**33**(32):3859−64.

71. Reece JC, Alcantara S, Gooneratne S, Jegaskanda S, Amaresena T, Fernandez CS, et al. Trivalent live attenuated influenza-SIV vaccines: efficacy and evolution of CTL escape in macaques. *J Virol* 2013.

72. Stebbings R, Fevrier M, Li B, Lorin C, Koutsoukos M, Mee E, et al. Immunogenicity of a recombinant measles-HIV-1 clade B candidate vaccine. *PLoS One* 2012;**7**(11):e50397.

73. Lorin C, Segal L, Mols J, Morelle D, Bourguignon P, Rovira O, et al. Toxicology, biodistribution and shedding profile of a recombinant measles vaccine vector expressing HIV-1 antigens, in cynomolgus macaques. *Naunyn-Schmiedeberg's Arch Pharmacol* 2012;**385** (12):1211−25.

74. Mourez T, Mesel-Lemoine M, Combredet C, Najburg V, Cayet N, Tangy F. A chimeric measles virus with a lentiviral envelope replicates exclusively in CD4+/CCR5+ cells. *Virology* 2011;**419**(2):117−25.

75. Xu R, Nasar F, Megati S, Luckay A, Lee M, Udem SA, et al. Prime-boost vaccination with recombinant mumps virus and recombinant vesicular stomatitis virus vectors elicits an enhanced human immunodeficiency virus type 1 Gag-specific cellular immune response in rhesus macaques. *J Virol* 2009;**83**(19):9813−23.

76. Carnero E, Li W, Borderia AV, Moltedo B, Moran T, Garcia-Sastre A. Optimization of human immunodeficiency virus gag expression by newcastle disease virus vectors for the induction of potent immune responses. *J Virol* 2009;**83**(2):584−97.

77. Khattar SK, Samal S, Devico AL, Collins PL, Samal SK. Newcastle disease virus expressing human immunodeficiency virus type 1 envelope glycoprotein induces strong mucosal and serum antibody responses in Guinea pigs. *J Virol* 2011;**85**(20):10529−41.

78. Maamary J, Array F, Gao Q, Garcia-Sastre A, Steinman RM, Palese P, et al. Newcastle disease virus expressing a dendritic cell-targeted HIV gag protein induces a potent gag-specific immune response in mice. *J Virol* 2011;**85**(5):2235−46.

79. McKenna PM, Koser ML, Carlson KR, Montefiori DC, Letvin NL, Papaneri AB, et al. Highly attenuated rabies virus-based vaccine vectors expressing simian-human immunodeficiency virus89.6P Env and simian immunodeficiency virusmac239 Gag are safe in rhesus macaques and protect from an AIDS-like disease. *J Infect Dis* 2007;**195**(7):980−8.

80. Faul EJ, Aye PP, Papaneri AB, Pahar B, McGettigan JP, Schiro F, et al. Rabies virus-based vaccines elicit neutralizing antibodies, poly-functional CD8 + T cell, and protect rhesus macaques from AIDS-like disease after SIV(mac251) challenge. *Vaccine* 2009;**28**(2): 299−308.

81. Matano T, Kobayashi M, Igarashi H, Takeda A, Nakamura H, Kano M, et al. Cytotoxic T lymphocyte-based control of simian immunodeficiency virus replication in a preclinical AIDS vaccine trial. *J Exp Med* 2004;**199**(12):1709−18.

82. Kawada M, Tsukamoto T, Yamamoto H, Takeda A, Igarashi H, Watkins DI, et al. Long-term control of simian immunodeficiency virus replication with central memory CD4+ T-cell preservation after nonsterile protection by a cytotoxic T-lymphocyte-based vaccine. *J Virol* 2007;**81**(10):5202−11.

83. Mayer AE, Johnson JB, Parks GD. The neutralizing capacity of antibodies elicited by parainfluenza virus infection of African Green Monkeys is dependent on complement. *Virology* 2014;**460-461**:23−33.

84. Rose NF, Marx PA, Luckay A, Nixon DF, Moretto WJ, Donahoe SM, et al. An effective AIDS vaccine based on live attenuated vesicular stomatitis virus recombinants. *Cell* 2001; **106**(5):539−49.

85. Rose NF, Roberts A, Buonocore L, Rose JK. Glycoprotein exchange vectors based on vesicular stomatitis virus allow effective boosting and generation of neutralizing antibodies to a primary isolate of human immunodeficiency virus type 1. *J Virol* 2000;**74**(23): 10903−10.

86. Cooper D, Wright KJ, Calderon PC, Guo M, Nasar F, Johnson JE, et al. Attenuation of recombinant vesicular stomatitis virus-human immunodeficiency virus type 1 vaccine vectors by gene translocations and g gene truncation reduces neurovirulence and enhances immunogenicity in mice. *J Virol* 2008;**82**(1):207−19.

87. Johnson JE, Coleman JW, Kalyan NK, Calderon P, Wright KJ, Obregon J, et al. In vivo biodistribution of a highly attenuated recombinant vesicular stomatitis virus expressing HIV-1 Gag following intramuscular, intranasal, or intravenous inoculation. *Vaccine* 2009;**27**(22):2930−9.

88. Jurgens CK, Morrow G, Boggiano C, Panis M, Coleman J, Powell R, et al. Evaluation of a replication-competent VSV-SIV vaccine candidate. *Retrovirology* 2012;**9**(Suppl. 2):P329.

89. Johnson JE, Schnell MJ, Buonocore L, Rose JK. Specific targeting to CD4+ cells of recombinant vesicular stomatitis viruses encoding human immunodeficiency virus envelope proteins. *J Virol* 1997;**71**(7):5060−8.

90. Deal C, Pekosz A, Ketner G. Prospects for oral replicating adenovirus-vectored vaccines. *Vaccine* 2013;**31**(32):3236−43.

91. Tuero I, Robert-Guroff M. Challenges in mucosal HIV vaccine development: lessons from non-human primate models. *Viruses* 2014;**6**(8):3129−58.

92. Priddy FH, Brown D, Kublin J, Monahan K, Wright DP, Lalezari J, et al. Safety and immunogenicity of a replication-incompetent adenovirus type 5 HIV-1 clade B gag/pol/ nef vaccine in healthy adults. *Clin Infect Dis* 2008;**46**(11):1769−81.

93. Catanzaro AT, Koup RA, Roederer M, Bailer RT, Enama ME, Moodie Z, et al. Phase 1 safety and immunogenicity evaluation of a multiclade HIV-1 candidate vaccine delivered by a replication-defective recombinant adenovirus vector. *J Infect Dis* 2006;**194**(12):1638−49.

94. Johnson JA, Barouch DH, Baden LR. Nonreplicating vectors in HIV vaccines. *Curr Opin HIV AIDS* 2013;**8**(5):412−20.

95. Gray G, Buchbinder S, Duerr A. Overview of STEP and Phambili trial results: two phase IIb test-of-concept studies investigating the efficacy of MRK adenovirus type 5 gag/pol/ nef subtype B HIV vaccine. *Curr Opin HIV AIDS* 2010;**5**(5):357−61.

96. Abbink P, Lemckert AA, Ewald BA, Lynch DM, Denholtz M, Smits S, et al. Comparative seroprevalence and immunogenicity of six rare serotype recombinant adenovirus vaccine vectors from subgroups B and D. *J Virol* 2007;**81**(9):4654−63.

97. Abbink P, Maxfield LF, Ng'ang'a D, Borducchi EN, Iampietro MJ, Bricault CA, et al. Construction and evaluation of novel rhesus monkey adenovirus vaccine vectors. *J Virol* 2015;**89**(3):1512−22.

98. Quinn KM, Da Costa A, Yamamoto A, Berry D, Lindsay RW, Darrah PA, et al. Comparative analysis of the magnitude, quality, phenotype, and protective capacity of simian immunodeficiency virus gag-specific CD8 + T cells following human-, simian-, and chimpanzee-derived recombinant adenoviral vector immunization. *J Immunol* 2013; **190**(6):2720−35.

99. Cervasi B, Carnathan DG, Sheehan KM, Micci L, Paiardini M, Kurupati R, et al. Immunological and virological analyses of rhesus macaques immunized with chimpanzee adenoviruses expressing the simian immunodeficiency virus Gag/Tat fusion protein and challenged intrarectally with repeated low doses of SIVmac. *J Virol* 2013;**87**(17): 9420−30.

100. Barouch DH. Novel adenovirus vector-based vaccines for HIV-1. *Curr Opin HIV AIDS* 2010;**5**(5):386−90.

101. Valentin A, McKinnon K, Li J, Rosati M, Kulkarni V, Pilkington GR, et al. Comparative analysis of SIV-specific cellular immune responses induced by different vaccine platforms in rhesus macaques. *Clin Immunol* 2014;**155**(1):91−107.

102. Arnberg N. Adenovirus receptors: implications for targeting of viral vectors. *Trends Pharmacol Sci* 2012;**33**(8):442−8.

103. Berk AJ. Adenoviridae. In: 6th ed. Knipe DM, Howley PM, editors. *Fields virology*, vol. 2. Philadelphia: Lippincott Williams and Wilkins; 2013. p. 1704−31.

104. Hendrickx R, Stichling N, Koelen J, Kuryk L, Lipiec A, Greber UF. Innate immunity to adenovirus. *Hum Gene Ther* 2014;**25**(4):265−84.

105. Bett AJ, Prevec L, Graham FL. Packaging capacity and stability of human adenovirus type 5 vectors. *J Virol* 1993;**67**(10):5911−21.

106. Wold WS, Toth K. Adenovirus vectors for gene therapy, vaccination and cancer gene therapy. *Curr Gene Ther* 2013;**13**(6):421−33.

107. Goncalves MA, de Vries AA. Adenovirus: from foe to friend. *Rev Med Virol* 2006;**16**(3): 167−86.

108. Alonso-Padilla J, Papp T, Kajan GL, Benko M, Havenga M, Lemckert A, et al. Development of Novel Adenoviral Vectors to Overcome Challenges Observed With HAdV-5-based Constructs. *Mol Ther* 2016;**24**(1):6−16.

109. Thomas MA, Song R, Demberg T, Vargas-Inchaustegui DA, Venzon D, Robert-Guroff M. Effects of the deletion of early region 4 (E4) open reading frame 1 (orf1), orf1-2, orf1-3 and orf1-4 on virus-host cell interaction, transgene expression, and immunogenicity of replicating adenovirus HIV vaccine vectors. *PLoS One* 2013;**8**(10):e76344.

110. Hoke Jr. CH, Snyder Jr. CE. History of the restoration of adenovirus type 4 and type 7 vaccine, live oral (Adenovirus Vaccine) in the context of the Department of Defense acquisition system. *Vaccine* 2013;**31**(12):1623−32.

111. Yun HC, Young AN, Caballero MY, Lott L, Cropper TL, Murray CK. Changes in clinical presentation and epidemiology of respiratory pathogens associated with acute respiratory illness in military trainees after reintroduction of adenovirus vaccine. *Open Forum Infect Dis* 2015;**2**(3):ofv120.

112. Barouch DH, Stephenson KE, Borducchi EN, Smith K, Stanley K, McNally AG, et al. Protective efficacy of a global HIV-1 mosaic vaccine against heterologous SHIV challenges in rhesus monkeys. *Cell* 2013;**155**(3):531−9.

113. Barouch DH, Liu J, Li H, Maxfield LF, Abbink P, Lynch DM, et al. Vaccine protection against acquisition of neutralization-resistant SIV challenges in rhesus monkeys. *Nature* 2012;**482**(7383):89−93.

114. Barouch DH, Alter G, Broge T, Linde C, Ackerman ME, Brown EP, et al. Protective efficacy of adenovirus/protein vaccines against SIV challenges in rhesus monkeys. *Science* 2015;**349**(6245):320−4.

115. Baden LR, Liu J, Li H, Johnson JA, Walsh SR, Kleinjan JA, et al. Induction of HIV-1-specific mucosal immune responses following intramuscular recombinant adenovirus serotype 26 HIV-1 vaccination of humans. *J Infect Dis* 2015;**211**(4):518−28.

116. Baden LR, Walsh SR, Seaman MS, Tucker RP, Krause KH, Patel A, et al. First-in-human evaluation of the safety and immunogenicity of a recombinant adenovirus serotype 26 HIV-1 Env vaccine (IPCAVD 001). *J Infect Dis* 2013;**207**(2):240−7.

117. Barouch DH, Liu J, Peter L, Abbink P, Iampietro MJ, Cheung A, et al. Characterization of humoral and cellular immune responses elicited by a recombinant adenovirus serotype 26 HIV-1 Env vaccine in healthy adults (IPCAVD 001). *J Infect Dis* 2013;**207**(2):248−56.

118. Crosby CM, Nehete P, Sastry KJ, Barry MA. Amplified and persistent immune responses generated by single-cycle replicating adenovirus vaccines. *J Virol* 2015;**89**(1):669−75.

119. Excler JL, Robb ML, Kim JH. HIV-1 vaccines: challenges and new perspectives. *Hum Vaccin Immunother* 2014;**10**(6):1734−46.

120. Lewis GK, DeVico AL, Gallo RC. Antibody persistence and T-cell balance: two key factors confronting HIV vaccine development. *Proc Natl Acad Sci USA* 2014;**111**(44):15614−21.

121. Bukh I, Calcedo R, Roy S, Carnathan DG, Grant R, Qin Q, et al. Increased mucosal CD4+ T cell activation in rhesus macaques following vaccination with an adenoviral vector. *J Virol* 2014;**88**(15):8468−78.

122. Carnathan DG, Wetzel KS, Yu J, Lee ST, Johnson BA, Paiardini M, et al. Activated CD4+ CCR5+ T cells in the rectum predict increased SIV acquisition in SIVGag/Tat-vaccinated rhesus macaques. *Proc Natl Acad Sci USA* 2015;**112**(2):518−23.

123. Pantaleo G, Esteban M, Jacobs B, Tartaglia J. Poxvirus vector-based HIV vaccines. *Curr Opin HIV AIDS* 2010;**5**(5):391−6.

124. Moss B. Reflections on the early development of poxvirus vectors. *Vaccine* 2013;**31**(39):4220−2.

125. Gomez CE, Perdiguero B, Garcia-Arriaza J, Esteban M. Poxvirus vectors as HIV/AIDS vaccines in humans. *Hum Vaccin Immunother* 2012;**8**(9):1192–207.
126. Paoletti E. Applications of pox virus vectors to vaccination: an update. *Proc Natl Acad Sci USA* 1996;**93**(21):11349–53.
127. Zhang Q, Tian M, Feng Y, Zhao K, Xu J, Liu Y, et al. Genomic sequence and virulence of clonal isolates of vaccinia virus Tiantan, the Chinese smallpox vaccine strain. *PLoS One* 2013;**8**(4):e60557.
128. Phanuphak N, Lo YR, Shao Y, Solomon SS, O'Connell RJ, Tovanabutra S, et al. HIV epidemic in Asia: implications for HIV vaccine and other prevention trials. *AIDS Res Hum Retroviruses* 2015.
129. Liu Q, Li Y, Luo Z, Yang G, Liu Y, Liu Y, et al. HIV-1 vaccines based on replication-competent Tiantan vaccinia protected Chinese rhesus macaques from simian HIV infection. *AIDS* 2015;**29**(6):649–58.
130. Smith GL, Benfield CT, Maluquer de Motes C, Mazzon M, Ember SW, Ferguson BJ, et al. Vaccinia virus immune evasion: mechanisms, virulence and immunogenicity. *J Gen Virol* 2013;**94**(Pt 11):2367–92.
131. Moss B. Poxviridae. In: Knipe DM, Howley PM, editors. *Fields virology*, vol. 2. Philadelphia: Lippincott Williams & Wilkins; 2013. p. 2129–59.
132. Sun C, Chen Z, Tang X, Zhang Y, Feng L, Du Y, et al. Mucosal prime with a replicating vaccinia-based vaccine elicits protective immunity against SIV challenge in rhesus monkeys. *J Virol* 2013.
133. Guo J, Zuo T, Cheng L, Wu X, Tang J, Sun C, et al. Simian immunodeficiency virus infection evades vaccine-elicited antibody responses to V2 region. *J Acquir Immune Defic Syndr* 2015;**68**(5):502–10.
134. Paoletti E, Tartaglia J, Taylor J. Safe and effective poxvirus vectors – NYVAC and ALVAC. *Dev Biol Stand* 1994;**82**:65–9.
135. Mooij P, Koopman G, Drijfhout JW, Nieuwenhuis IG, Beenhakker N, Koestler J, et al. Synthetic long peptide booster immunization in rhesus macaques primed with replication-competent NYVAC-C-KC induces a balanced CD4/CD8 T-cell and antibody response against the conserved regions of HIV-1. *J Gen Virol* 2015;**96**(Pt 6):1478–83.
136. Heeney JL, Jacobs B, Esteban M, Wagner R, Foulds K, Roederer M, et al. Increased HIV-1 immunogenicity of replication competent NYVAC. *AIDS Res Hum Retroviruses* 2013;**29**(11). A160-A.
137. Pellett PE, Roizman B. Herpesviridae. In: Knipe DM, Howley PM, editors. *Fields virology*, vol. 2. Philadelphia: Lippincott Williams and Wilkins; 2013. p. 1802–22.
138. Moore PL, Williamson C, Morris L. Virological features associated with the development of broadly neutralizing antibodies to HIV-1. *Trends Microbiol* 2015;**23**(4):204–11.
139. Shin YC, Bischof GF, Lauer WA, Desrosiers RC. Importance of codon usage for the temporal regulation of viral gene expression. *Proc Natl Acad Sci USA* 2015.
140. Mocarski ES, Shenk T, Griffiths PD, Pass RF. Cytomegaloviruses. In: Knipe DM, Howley PM, editors. *Fields virology*, vol. 2. Philadelphia: Lippincott Williams and Wilkins; 2013. p. 1960–2014.
141. Britt W. Manifestations of human cytomegalovirus infection: proposed mechanisms of acute and chronic disease. *Curr Top Microbiol Immunol* 2008;**325**:417–70.
142. Chang WL, Barry PA. Cloning of the full-length rhesus cytomegalovirus genome as an infectious and self-excisable bacterial artificial chromosome for analysis of viral pathogenesis. *J Virol* 2003;**77**(9):5073–83.

143. Malouli D, Nakayasu ES, Viswanathan K, Camp 2nd DG, Chang WL, Barry PA, et al. Reevaluation of the coding potential and proteomic analysis of the BAC-derived rhesus cytomegalovirus strain 68-1. *J Virol* 2012;**86**(17):8959−73.

144. Hansen SG, Strelow LI, Franchi DC, Anders DG, Wong SW. Complete sequence and genomic analysis of rhesus cytomegalovirus. *J Virol* 2003;**77**(12):6620−36.

145. Hansen SG, Piatak Jr. M, Ventura AB, Hughes CM, Gilbride RM, Ford JC, et al. Immune clearance of highly pathogenic SIV infection. *Nature* 2013;**502**(7469):100−4.

146. Picker LJ. Are effector memory T cells the key to an effective HIV/AIDS vaccine? *EMBO Rep* 2014;**15**(8):820−1.

147. Barouch DH, Picker LJ. Novel vaccine vectors for HIV-1. *Nat Rev Microbiol* 2014;**12**(11):765−71.

148. Hansen SG, Sacha JB, Hughes CM, Ford JC, Burwitz BJ, Scholz I, et al. Cytomegalovirus vectors violate CD8+ T cell epitope recognition paradigms. *Science* 2013;**340**(6135):1237874.

149. Ranasinghe S, Walker BD. Programming CMV for vaccine vector design. *Nat Biotechnol* 2013;**31**(9):811−12.

150. Murphy E, Shenk T. Human cytomegalovirus genome. *Curr Top Microbiol Immunol* 2008;**325**:1−19.

151. Davison AJ, Dolan A, Akter P, Addison C, Dargan DJ, Alcendor DJ, et al. The human cytomegalovirus genome revisited: comparison with the chimpanzee cytomegalovirus genome. *J Gen Virol* 2003;**84**(Pt 1):17−28.

152. Pereira L, Maidji E. Cytomegalovirus infection in the human placenta: maternal immunity and developmentally regulated receptors on trophoblasts converge. *Curr Top Microbiol Immunol* 2008;**325**:383−95.

153. Krause PR, Bialek SR, Boppana SB, Griffiths PD, Laughlin CA, Ljungman P, et al. Priorities for CMV vaccine development. *Vaccine* 2013;**32**(1):4−10.

154. Heineman TC, Schleiss M, Bernstein DI, Spaete RR, Yan L, Duke G, et al. A phase 1 study of 4 live, recombinant human cytomegalovirus Towne/Toledo chimeric vaccines. *J Infect Dis* 2006;**193**(10):1350−60.

155. Malouli D, Hansen SG, Nakayasu ES, Marshall EE, Hughes CM, Ventura AB, et al. Cytomegalovirus pp65 limits dissemination but is dispensable for persistence. *J Clin Invest* 2014;**124**(5):1928−44.

156. Estep RD, Wong SW. Rhesus macaque rhadinovirus-associated disease. *Curr Opin Virol* 2013;**3**(3):245−50.

157. Fukazawa Y, Park H, Cameron MJ, Lefebvre F, Lum R, Coombes N, et al. Lymph node T cell responses predict the efficacy of live attenuated SIV vaccines. *Nat Med* 2012;**18**(11):1673−81.

158. Bilello JP, Morgan JS, Desrosiers RC. Extreme dependence of gH and gL expression on ORF57 and association with highly unusual codon usage in rhesus monkey rhadinovirus. *J Virol* 2008;**82**(14):7231−7.

159. Shin YC, Desrosiers RC. Rhesus monkey rhadinovirus ORF57 induces gH and gL glycoprotein expression through posttranscriptional accumulation of target mRNAs. *J Virol* 2011;**85**(15):7810−17.

160. Ouwendijk WJ, Laing KJ, Verjans GM, Koelle DM. T-cell immunity to human alphaher-pesviruses. *Curr Opin Virol* 2013;**3**(4):452−60.

161. Gershon AA. Varicella zoster vaccines and their implications for development of HSV vaccines. *Virology* 2013;**435**(1):29−36.

162. Takahashi M, Asano Y, Kamiya H, Baba K, Ozaki T, Otsuka T, et al. Development of varicella vaccine. *J Infect Dis* 2008;**197**(Suppl. 2):S41−4.

163. Murakami K, Mori Y. Use of a current varicella vaccine as a live polyvalent vaccine vector. *Vaccine* 2014.

164. Gray WL. Recombinant varicella-zoster virus vaccines as platforms for expression of foreign antigens. *Adv Virol* 2013;**2013**:219439.

165. Ouwendijk WJ, Verjans GM. Pathogenesis of varicelloviruses in primates. *J Pathol* 2015; **235**(2):298−311.

166. Meyer C, Engelmann F, Arnold N, Krah DL, ter Meulen J, Haberthur K, et al. Abortive intrabronchial infection of rhesus macaques with varicella-zoster virus provides partial protection against simian varicella virus challenge. *J Virol* 2015;**89**(3):1781−93.

167. Staprans SI, Barry AP, Silvestri G, Safrit JT, Kozyr N, Sumpter B, et al. Enhanced SIV replication and accelerated progression to AIDS in macaques primed to mount a CD4 T cell response to the SIV envelope protein. *Proc Natl Acad Sci USA* 2004;**101**(35): 13026−31.

168. Traina-Dorge V, Pahar B, Marx P, Kissinger P, Montefiori D, Ou Y, et al. Recombinant varicella vaccines induce neutralizing antibodies and cellular immune responses to SIV and reduce viral loads in immunized rhesus macaques. *Vaccine* 2010;**28**(39):6483−90.

169. Veterinary Biological Products [Internet]. Center for Veterinary Biologics Policy, Evaluation, and Licensing. Available from: https://www.aphis.usda.gov/animal_health/ vet_biologics/publications/CurrentProdCodeBook.pdf; 2015 [cited 10.11.15].

170. Rayner JO, Dryga SA, Kamrud KI. Alphavirus vectors and vaccination. *Rev Med Virol* 2002;**12**(5):279−96.

171. Almazan F, Sola I, Zuniga S, Marquez-Jurado S, Morales L, Becares M, et al. Coronavirus reverse genetic systems: infectious clones and replicons. *Virus Res* 2014;**189**: 262−70.

172. Geall AJ, Mandl CW, Ulmer JB. RNA: the new revolution in nucleic acid vaccines. *Semin Immunol* 2013;**25**(2):152−9.

173. Racaniello VR. Picornaviridae: the viruses and their replication. In: Knipe DM, Howley PM, editors. *Fields virology*, vol. 1. Philadelphia: Lippincott Williams and Wilkins; 2013. p. 453−89.

174. Kuhn RJ. Togaviridae. In: Knipe DM, Howley PM, editors. *Fields virology*, vol. 1. Philadelphia: Lippincott Williams and Wilkins; 2013. p. 629−50.

175. Lindenbach BD, Murray CL, Heinz-Jurgens T, Rice CM. Flaviviridae. In: Knipe DM, Howley PM, editors. *Fields virology*, vol. 1. Philadelphia: Lippincott Williams and Wilkins; 2013. p. 712−46.

176. Monath TP. Yellow fever vaccine. *Expert Rev Vaccines* 2005;**4**(4):553−74.

177. Bonaldo MC, Sequeira PC, Galler R. The yellow fever 17D virus as a platform for new live attenuated vaccines. *Hum Vaccin Immunother* 2014;**10**(5):1256−65.

178. Galler R, Freire MS, Jabor AV, Mann GF. The yellow fever 17D vaccine virus: molecular basis of viral attenuation and its use as an expression vector. *Braz J Med Biol Res* 1997; **30**(2):157−68.

179. De Santana MG, Neves PC, dos Santos JR, Lima NS, dos Santos AA, Watkins DI, et al. Improved genetic stability of recombinant yellow fever 17D virus expressing a lentiviral Gag gene fragment. *Virology* 2014;**452-453**:202−11.

180. Franco D, Li W, Qing F, Stoyanov CT, Moran T, Rice CM, et al. Evaluation of yellow fever virus 17D strain as a new vector for HIV-1 vaccine development. *Vaccine* 2010;**28** (35):5676−85.

181. Martins MA, Tully DC, Cruz MA, Power KA, Veloso de Santana MG, Bean DJ, et al. Vaccine-Induced Simian Immunodeficiency Virus-Specific CD8 + T-Cell Responses Focused on a Single Nef Epitope Select for Escape Variants Shortly after Infection. *J Virol* 2015;**89**(21):10802−20.

182. Martins MA, Wilson NA, Piaskowski SM, Weisgrau KL, Furlott JR, Bonaldo MC, et al. Vaccination with Gag, Vif, and Nef gene fragments affords partial control of viral replication after mucosal challenge with SIVmac239. *J Virol* 2014;**88**(13):7493−516.

183. Martins MA, Wilson NA, Reed JS, Ahn CD, Klimentidis YC, Allison DB, et al. T-cell correlates of vaccine efficacy after a heterologous simian immunodeficiency virus challenge. *J Virol* 2010;**84**(9):4352−65.

184. Virnik K, Hockenbury M, Ni Y, Beren J, Pavlakis GN, Felber BK, et al. Live attenuated rubella vectors expressing SIV and HIV vaccine antigens replicate and elicit durable immune responses in rhesus macaques. *Retrovirology* 2013;**10**:99.

185. Virnik K, Ni Y, Berkower I. Enhanced expression of HIV and SIV vaccine antigens in the structural gene region of live attenuated rubella viral vectors and their incorporation into virions. *Vaccine* 2013.

186. Rosati M, Alicea C, Kulkarni V, Virnik K, Hockenbury M, Sardesai NY, et al. Recombinant rubella vectors elicit SIV Gag-specific T cell responses with cytotoxic potential in rhesus macaques. *Vaccine* 2015;**33**(18):2167−74.

187. Rose NF, Buonocore L, Schell JB, Chattopadhyay A, Bahl K, Liu X, et al. In vitro evolution of high-titer, virus-like vesicles containing a single structural protein. *Proc Natl Acad Sci USA* 2014;**111**(47):16866−71.

188. Schell JB, Bahl K, Folta-Stogniew E, Rose N, Buonocore L, Marx PA, et al. Antigenic requirement for Gag in a vaccine that protects against high-dose mucosal challenge with simian immunodeficiency virus. *Virology* 2015;**476**:405−12.

189. Gambhira R, Keele BF, Schell JB, Hunter MJ, Dufour JP, Montefiori DC, et al. Transmitted/founder simian immunodeficiency virus envelope sequences in vesicular stomatitis and Semliki forest virus vector immunized rhesus macaques. *PLoS One* 2014;**9**(10):e109678.

190. Yi G, Lapelosa M, Bradley R, Mariano TM, Dietz DE, Hughes S, et al. Chimeric rhinoviruses displaying MPER epitopes elicit anti-HIV neutralizing responses. *PLoS One* 2013;**8**(9):e72205.

191. Yi G, Tu X, Bharaj P, Guo H, Zhang J, Shankar P, et al. Human rhinovirus presenting 4E10 epitope of HIV-1 MPER elicits neutralizing antibodies in human ICAM-1 transgenic mice. *Mol Ther* 2015;**23**(10):1663−70.

192. Tomusange K, Yu W, Suhrbier A, Wijesundara D, Grubor-Bauk B, Gowans EJ. Engineering human rhinovirus serotype-A1 as a vaccine vector. *Virus Res* 2015;**203**:72−6.

193. Clarke E, Desselberger U. Correlates of protection against human rotavirus disease and the factors influencing protection in low-income settings. *Mucosal Immunol* 2015;**8**(1):1−17.

194. Dermody TS, Parker JSL, Sherry B. Orthoreoviruses. In: Knipe DM, Howley PM, editors. *Fields virology*, vol. 2. Philadelphia: Lippincott Williams and Wilkins; 2013. p. 1304−46.

195. Kobayashi T, Antar AA, Boehme KW, Danthi P, Eby EA, Guglielmi KM, et al. A plasmid-based reverse genetics system for animal double-stranded RNA viruses. *Cell Host Microbe* 2007;**1**(2):147−57.

196. Tai JH, Williams JV, Edwards KM, Wright PF, Crowe Jr. JE, Dermody TS. Prevalence of reovirus-specific antibodies in young children in Nashville, Tennessee. *J Infect Dis* 2005;**191**(8):1221−4.

197. Bukreyev A, Skiadopoulos MH, Murphy BR, Collins PL. Nonsegmented negative-strand viruses as vaccine vectors. *J Virol* 2006;**80**(21):10293—306.

198. Pfaller CK, Cattaneo R, Schnell MJ. Reverse genetics of Mononegavirales: how they work, new vaccines, and new cancer therapeutics. *Virology* 2015;**479—480**:331—44.

199. Buczkowski H, Muniraju M, Parida S, Banyard AC. Morbillivirus vaccines: recent successes and future hopes. *Vaccine* 2014;**32**(26):3155—61.

200. Ellis JA. Bovine parainfluenza-3 virus. *Vet Clin North Am Food Anim Pract* 2010;**26**(3): 575—93.

201. Alexander DJ, Senne DA. Newcastle disease, other avain paramyxoviruses, and pneumo-virus infections. In: Saif YM, Fadly AM, Glisson JR, McDougald LR, Nolan LK, Swayne DE, editors. *Diseases of poultry*. 12th ed. Ames, Iowa, United States: Blackwell Publishing; 2008. p. 75—100.

202. Conzelmann KK. Reverse genetics of mononcgavirales. *Curr Top Microbiol Immunol* 2004;**283**:1—41.

203. Neumann G, Whitt MA, Kawaoka Y. A decade after the generation of a negative-sense RNA virus from cloned cDNA — what have we learned? *J Gen Virol* 2002;**83**(Pt 11): 2635—62.

204. Billeter MA, Naim HY, Udem SA. Reverse genetics of measles virus and resulting multi-valent recombinant vaccines: applications of recombinant measles viruses. *Curr Top Microbiol Immunol* 2009;**329**:129—62.

205. Johnson JE, Nasar F, Coleman JW, Price RE, Javadian A, Draper K, et al. Neurovirulence properties of recombinant vesicular stomatitis virus vectors in non-human primates. *Virology* 2007;**360**(1):36—49.

206. Clarke DK, Nasar F, Chong S, Johnson JE, Coleman JW, Lee M, et al. Neurovirulence and immunogenicity of attenuated recombinant vesicular stomatitis viruses in nonhuman primates. *J Virol* 2014;**88**(12):6690—701.

207. Fuchs JD, Frank I, Elizaga ML, Allen M, Frahm N, Kochar N, et al. First-in-human evaluation of the safety and immunogenicity of a recombinant vesicular stomatitis virus human immunodeficiency virus-1 gag vaccine (HVTN 090). *Open Forum Infect Dis* 2015;**2**(3):ofv082.

208. Egan MA, Chong SY, Megati S, Montefiori DC, Rose NF, Boyer JD, et al. Priming with plasmid DNAs expressing interleukin-12 and simian immunodeficiency virus gag enhances the immunogenicity and efficacy of an experimental AIDS vaccine based on recombinant vesicular stomatitis virus. *AIDS Res Hum Retroviruses* 2005;**21**(7):629—43.

209. Hay CM, Wilson GJ, Elizaga M, Li S, Kochar N, Tomoras GD, et al. An HIV DNA vaccine delivered by electroporation and boosted by rVSV HIV-1 Gag is safe and immu-no- genic in healthy HIV-uninfected adults. HIV Research for Prevention 2014: AIDS Vaccine, Microbicide, and ARV-based Prevention Science (HIV R4P); October 28; Cape Town, South Africa: AIDS Research and Human Retroviruses; 2014. p. A17.

210. Marthas ML, Van Rompay KK, Abbott Z, Earl P, Buonocore-Buzzelli L, Moss B, et al. Partial efficacy of a VSV-SIV/MVA-SIV vaccine regimen against oral SIV challenge in infant macaques. *Vaccine* 2011;**29**(17):3124—37.

211. Van Rompay KK, Abel K, Earl P, Kozlowski PA, Easlick J, Moore J, et al. Immunogenicity of viral vector, prime-boost SIV vaccine regimens in infant rhesus maca-ques: attenuated vesicular stomatitis virus (VSV) and modified vaccinia Ankara (MVA) recombinant SIV vaccines compared to live-attenuated SIV. *Vaccine* 2010;**28**(6): 1481—92.

212. Schell J, Rose NF, Fazo N, Marx PA, Hunter M, Ramsburg E, et al. Long-term vaccine protection from AIDS and clearance of viral DNA following SHIV89.6P challenge. *Vaccine* 2009;**27**(7):979–86.

213. Rabinovich S, Powell RL, Lindsay RW, Yuan M, Carpov A, Wilson A, et al. A novel, live-attenuated vesicular stomatitis virus vector displaying conformationally intact, functional HIV-1 envelope trimers that elicits potent cellular and humoral responses in mice. *PLoS One* 2014;**9**(9):e106597.

214. Lorenz IC, Nguyen HT, Kemelman M, Lindsay RW, Yuan M, Wright KJ, et al. The stem of vesicular stomatitis virus G can be replaced with the HIV-1 Env membrane-proximal external region without loss of G function or membrane-proximal external region antigenic properties. *AIDS Res Hum Retroviruses* 2014;**30**(11):1130–44.

215. Wu K, Kim GN, Kang CY. Expression and processing of human immunodeficiency virus type 1 gp160 using the vesicular stomatitis virus New Jersey serotype vector system. *J Gen Virol* 2009;**90**(Pt 5):1135–40.

216. Schlehuber LD, Rose JK. Prediction and identification of a permissive epitope insertion site in the vesicular stomatitis virus glycoprotein. *J Virol* 2004;**78**(10):5079–87.

217. Lawrence TM, Wanjalla CN, Gomme EA, Wirblich C, Gatt A, Carnero E, et al. Comparison of heterologous prime-boost strategies against human immunodeficiency virus type 1 Gag using negative stranded RNA viruses. *PLoS One* 2013;**8**(6):e67123.

218. McGettigan JP, Pomerantz RJ, Siler CA, McKenna PM, Foley HD, Dietzschold B, et al. Second-generation rabies virus-based vaccine vectors expressing human immunodeficiency virus type 1 gag have greatly reduced pathogenicity but are highly immunogenic. *J Virol* 2003;**77**(1):237–44.

219. Mebatsion T, Weiland F, Conzelmann KK. Matrix protein of rabies virus is responsible for the assembly and budding of bullet-shaped particles and interacts with the transmembrane spike glycoprotein G. *J Virol* 1999;**73**(1):242–50.

220. Dunkel A, Shen S, LaBranche CC, Montefiori D, McGettigan JP. A bivalent, chimeric rabies virus expressing simian immunodeficiency virus envelope induces multifunctional antibody responses. *AIDS Res Hum Retroviruses* 2015.

221. Faisca P, Desmecht D. Sendai virus, the mouse parainfluenza type 1: a longstanding pathogen that remains up-to-date. *Res Vet Sci* 2007;**82**(1):115–25.

222. Ishii H, Matano T. Development of an AIDS vaccine using Sendai virus vectors. *Vaccine* 2015.

223. Hara H, Hara H, Hironaka T, Inoue M, Iida A, Shu T, et al. Prevalence of specific neutralizing antibodies against Sendai virus in populations from different geographic areas: implications for AIDS vaccine development using Sendai virus vectors. *Hum Vaccin* 2011;**7**(6):639–45.

224. Moriya C, Horiba S, Kurihara K, Kamada T, Takahara Y, Inoue M, et al. Intranasal Sendai viral vector vaccination is more immunogenic than intramuscular under pre-existing anti-vector antibodies. *Vaccine* 2011;**29**(47):8557–63.

225. Keefer MC, Gilmour J, Hayes P, Gill D, Kopycinski J, Cheeseman H, et al. A phase I double blind, placebo-controlled, randomized study of a multigenic HIV-1 adenovirus subtype 35 vector vaccine in healthy uninfected adults. *PLoS One* 2012;**7**(8):e41936.

226. Karita E, Anzala O, Gazzard. B, Bergin P, Nyombayire J, Omosa G, et al. Clinical safety and immunogenicity of two HIV vaccines SeV-G (NP) and Ad35-GRIN in HIV-uninfected, healthy adult volunteers. October 30, 2014; Cape Twon, South Africa: AIDS Research and Human Retroviruses; 2014.

227. Ganar K, Das M, Sinha S, Kumar S. Newcastle disease virus: current status and our understanding. *Virus Res* 2014;**184**:71−81.

228. Bukreyev A, Collins PL. Newcastle disease virus as a vaccine vector for humans. *Curr Opin Mol Ther* 2008;**10**(1):46−55.

229. Cuadrado-Castano S, Sanchez-Aparicio MT, Garcia-Sastre A, Villar E. The therapeutic effect of death: Newcastle disease virus and its antitumor potential. *Virus Res* 2015.

230. Fournier P, Schirrmacher V. Oncolytic newcastle disease virus as cutting edge between tumor and host. *Biology (Basel)* 2013;**2**(3):936−75.

231. Zamarin D, Pesonen S. Replication-competent viruses as cancer immunotherapeutics: emerging clinical data. *Hum Gene Ther* 2015;**26**(8):538−49.

232. Nakaya Y, Nakaya T, Park MS, Cros J, Imanishi J, Palese P, et al. Induction of cellular immune responses to simian immunodeficiency virus gag by two recombinant negative-strand RNA virus vectors. *J Virol* 2004;**78**(17):9366−75.

233. Khattar SK, Samal S, LaBranche CC, Montefiori DC, Collins PL, Samal SK. Comparative immunogenicity of HIV-1 gp160, gp140 and gp120 expressed by live attenuated newcastle disease virus vector. *PLoS One* 2013;**8**(10):e78521.

234. Khattar SK, Palaniyandi S, Samal S, LaBranche CC, Montefiori DC, Zhu X, et al. Evaluation of humoral, mucosal, and cellular immune responses following co-immunization of HIV-1 Gag and Env proteins expressed by Newcastle disease virus. *Hum Vaccin Immunother* 2015;**11**(2):504−15.

235. Khattar SK, Manoharan V, Bhattarai B, LaBranche CC, Montefiori DC, Samal SK. Mucosal immunization with Newcastle disease virus vector coexpressing HIV-1 Env and Gag proteins elicits potent serum, mucosal, and cellular immune responses that protect against vaccinia virus Env and Gag challenges. *mBio* 2015;**6**(4):e01005.

236. Lievano F, Galea SA, Thornton M, Wiedmann RT, Manoff SB, Tran TN, et al. Measles, mumps, and rubella virus vaccine (M-M-RII): a review of 32 years of clinical and postmarketing experience. *Vaccine* 2012;**30**(48):6918−26.

237. Rima BK, Gatherer D, Young DF, Norsted H, Randall RE, Davison AJ. Stability of the parainfluenza virus 5 genome revealed by deep sequencing of strains isolated from different hosts and following passage in cell culture. *J Virol* 2014;**88**(7):3826−36.

238. De Vries RD, Duprex WP, de Swart RL. Morbillivirus infections: an introduction. *Viruses* 2015;**7**(2):699−706.

239. Bankamp B, Takeda M, Zhang Y, Xu W, Rota PA. Genetic characterization of measles vaccine strains. *J Infect Dis* 2011;**204**(Suppl. 1):S533−48.

240. Martella V, Elia G, Buonavoglia C. Canine distemper virus. *Vet Clin North Am Small Anim Pract* 2008;**38**(4):787−97, vii−viii.

241. De Vries RD, Lemon K, Ludlow M, McQuaid S, Yuksel S, van Amerongen G, et al. In vivo tropism of attenuated and pathogenic measles virus expressing green fluorescent protein in macaques. *J Virol* 2010;**84**(9):4714−24.

242. Von Messling V, Milosevic D, Cattaneo R. Tropism illuminated: lymphocyte-based pathways blazed by lethal morbillivirus through the host immune system. *Proc Natl Acad Sci USA* 2004;**101**(39):14216−21.

243. Fukazawa Y, Lum R, Okoye AA, Park H, Matsuda K, Bae JY, et al. B cell follicle sanctuary permits persistent productive simian immunodeficiency virus infection in elite controllers. *Nat. Med.* 2015;**21**(2):132−9.

244. Ferguson D, Mattiuzzo G, Ham C, Stebbings R, Li B, Rose NJ, et al. Early biodistribution and persistence of a protective live attenuated SIV vaccine elicits localised innate responses in multiple lymphoid tissues. *PLoS One* 2014;**9**(8):e104390.

245. Rennick LJ, de Vries RD, Carsillo TJ, Lemon K, van Amerongen G, Ludlow M, et al. Live-attenuated measles virus vaccine targets dendritic cells and macrophages in muscle of nonhuman primates. *J Virol* 2015;**89**(4):2192−200.

246. Lin WH, Kouyos RD, Adams RJ, Grenfell BT, Griffin DE. Prolonged persistence of measles virus RNA is characteristic of primary infection dynamics. *Proc Natl Acad Sci USA* 2012;**109**(37):14989−94.

247. Stebbings R, Li B, Lorin C, Koutsoukos M, Fevrier M, Mee ET, et al. Immunogenicity of a recombinant measles HIV-1 subtype C vaccine. *Vaccine* 2013;**31**(51):6079−86.

248. Chen RT, Markowitz LE, Albrecht P, Stewart JA, Mofenson LM, Preblud SR, et al. Measles antibody: reevaluation of protective titers. *J Infect Dis* 1990;**162**(5):1036−42.

249. Dine MS, Hutchins SS, Thomas A, Williams I, Bellini WJ, Redd SC. Persistence of vaccine-induced antibody to measles 26−33 years after vaccination. *J Infect Dis* 2004;**189**(Suppl. 1):S123−30.

250. Croyle MA, Patel A, Tran KN, Gray M, Zhang Y, Strong JE, et al. Nasal delivery of an adenovirus-based vaccine bypasses pre-existing immunity to the vaccine carrier and improves the immune response in mice. *PLoS One* 2008;**3**(10):e3548.

251. Knuchel MC, Marty RR, Morin TN, Ilter O, Zuniga A, Naim HY. Relevance of a pre-existing measles immunity prior immunization with a recombinant measles virus vector. *Hum Vaccin Immunother* 2013;**9**(3):599−606.

252. Miest TS, Yaiw KC, Frenzke M, Lampe J, Hudacek AW, Springfeld C, et al. Envelope-chimeric entry-targeted measles virus escapes neutralization and achieves oncolysis. *Mol Ther* 2011;**19**(10):1813−20.

253. Hudacek AW, Navaratnarajah CK, Cattaneo R. Development of measles virus-based shielded oncolytic vectors: suitability of other paramyxovirus glycoproteins. *Cancer Gene Ther* 2013;**20**(2):109−16.

254. Spielhofer P, Bachi T, Fehr T, Christiansen G, Cattaneo R, Kaelin K, et al. Chimeric measles viruses with a foreign envelope. *J Virol* 1998;**72**(3):2150−9.

255. Zhang X, Wallace OL, Domi A, Wright KJ, Driscoll J, Anzala O, et al. Canine distemper virus neutralization activity is low in human serum and it is sensitive to an amino acid substitution in the hemagglutinin protein. *Virology* 2015;**482**:218−24.

256. Rima BK, Duprex WP. Morbilliviruses and human disease. *J Pathol* 2006;**208**(2):199−214.

257. Haig DA. Canine distemper-immunisation with avianized virus. *Onderstepoort J Vet Res* 1956;**27**(1):19−53.

258. Hoekenga MT, Schwarz AJ, Carrizo Palma H, Boyer PA. Experimental vaccination against measles. II. Tests of live measles and live distemper vaccine in human volunteers during a measles epidemic in Panama. *J Am Med Assoc* 1960;**173**:868−72.

259. Schwarz AJ, Boyer PA, Zirbel LW, York CJ. Experimental vaccination against measles. I. Tests of live measles and distemper vaccine in monkeys and two human volunteers under laboratory conditions. *J Am Med Assoc* 1960;**173**:861−7.

260. Jin H, Subbarao K. Live attenuated influenza vaccine. *Curr Top Microbiol Immunol* 2015;**386**:181−204.

261. Ambrose CS, Levin MJ, Belshe RB. The relative efficacy of trivalent live attenuated and inactivated influenza vaccines in children and adults. *Influenza Other Respir Viruses* 2011;**5**(2):67−75.

262. Ozawa M, Kawaoka Y. Taming influenza viruses. *Virus Res* 2011;**162**(1−2):8−11.

263. Goto H, Muramoto Y, Noda T, Kawaoka Y. The genome-packaging signal of the influenza A virus genome comprises a genome incorporation signal and a genome-bundling signal. *J Virol* 2013;**87**(21):11316−22.

264. Garulli B, Di Mario G, Stillitano MG, Compagnoni D, Titti F, Cafaro A, et al. Induction of antibodies and T cell responses by a recombinant influenza virus carrying an HIV-1 TatDelta51-59 protein in mice. *Biomed Res Int* 2014;**2014**:904038.

265. Garulli B, Di Mario G, Stillitano MG, Kawaoka Y, Castrucci MR. Exploring mucosal immunization with a recombinant influenza virus carrying an HIV-polyepitope in mice with pre-existing immunity to influenza. *Vaccine* 2014;**32**(21):2501−6.

266. Sexton A, De Rose R, Reece JC, Alcantara S, Loh L, Moffat JM, et al. Evaluation of recombinant influenza virus-simian immunodeficiency virus vaccines in macaques. *J Virol* 2009;**83**(15):7619−28.

267. Torresi J, McCarthy K, Feroldi E, Meric C. Immunogenicity, safety and tolerability in adults of a new single-dose, live-attenuated vaccine against Japanese encephalitis: randomised controlled phase 3 trials. *Vaccine* 2010;**28**(50):7993−8000.

268. Jones SM, Feldmann H, Stroher U, Geisbert JB, Fernando L, Grolla A, et al. Live attenuated recombinant vaccine protects nonhuman primates against Ebola and Marburg viruses. *Nature medicine* 2005;**11**(7):786−90.

269. Regules JA, Beigel JH, Paolino KM, Voell J, Castellano AR, Munoz P, et al. A Recombinant vesicular stomatitis virus ebola vaccine-preliminary report. *N Eng J Med* 2015.

270. Henao-Restrepo AM, Longini IM, Egger M, Dean NE, Edmunds WJ, Camacho A, et al. Efficacy and effectiveness of an rVSV-vectored vaccine expressing Ebola surface glycoprotein: interim results from the Guinea ring vaccination cluster-randomised trial. *Lancet* 2015;**386**(9996):857−66.

271. Agnandji ST, Huttner A, Zinser ME, Njuguna P, Dahlke C, Fernandes JF, et al. Phase 1 trials of rVSV ebola vaccine in Africa and Europe-preliminary report. *N Eng J Med* 2015.

272. Huttner A, Dayer JA, Yerly S, Combescure C, Auderset F, Desmeules J, et al. The effect of dose on the safety and immunogenicity of the VSV Ebola candidate vaccine: a randomised double-blind, placebo-controlled phase 1/2 trial. *Lancet Infect Dis* 2015;**15**(10):1156−66.

273. Boritz E, Gerlach J, Johnson JE, Rose JK. Replication-competent rhabdoviruses with human immunodeficiency virus type 1 coats and green fluorescent protein: entry by a pH-independent pathway. *J Virol* 1999;**73**(8):6937−45.

274. Mire CE, Miller AD, Carville A, Westmoreland SV, Geisbert JB, Mansfield KG, et al. Recombinant vesicular stomatitis virus vaccine vectors expressing filovirus glycoproteins lack neurovirulence in nonhuman primates. *PLoS Negl Trop Dis* 2012;**6**(3):e1567.

275. Wollmann G, Drokhlyansky E, Davis JN, Cepko C, van den Pol AN. Lassa-vesicular stomatitis chimeric virus safely destroys brain tumors. *J Virol* 2015;**89**(13):6711−24.

276. Muik A, Stubbert LJ, Jahedi RZ, Geibeta Y, Kimpel J, Dold C, et al. Re-engineering vesicular stomatitis virus to abrogate neurotoxicity, circumvent humoral immunity, and enhance oncolytic potency. *Cancer Res* 2014;**74**(13):3567−78.

277. Khalil SM, Tonkin DR, Snead AT, Parks GD, Johnston RE, White LJ. An alphavirus-based adjuvant enhances serum and mucosal antibodies, T cells, and protective immunity to influenza virus in neonatal mice. *J Virol* 2014;**88**(16):9182−96.

278. Steil BP, Jorquera P, Westdijk J, Bakker WA, Johnston RE, Barro M. A mucosal adjuvant for the inactivated poliovirus vaccine. *Vaccine* 2014;**32**(5):558−63.

279. Dalgleish AG, Beverley PC, Clapham PR, Crawford DH, Greaves MF, Weiss RA. The CD4 (T4) antigen is an essential component of the receptor for the AIDS retrovirus. *Nature* 1984;**312**(5996):763−7.

280. Owens RJ, Rose JK. Cytoplasmic domain requirement for incorporation of a foreign envelope protein into vesicular stomatitis virus. *J Virol* 1993;**67**(1):360−5.

281. Johnson JE, Rodgers W, Rose JK. A plasma membrane localization signal in the HIV-1 envelope cytoplasmic domain prevents localization at sites of vesicular stomatitis virus budding and incorporation into VSV virions. *Virology* 1998;**251**(2):244−52.

282. Horvath CM. Weapons of STAT destruction. Interferon evasion by paramyxovirus V protein. *Eur J Biochem/FEBS* 2004;**271**(23−24):4621−8.

283. Rieder M, Conzelmann KK. Rhabdovirus evasion of the interferon system. *J Interferon Cytokine Res* 2009;**29**(9):499−509.

284. Weitzman MD, Ornelles DA. Inactivating intracellular antiviral responses during adenovirus infection. *Oncogene* 2005;**24**(52):7686−96.

285. Powers C, DeFilippis V, Malouli D, Fruh K. Cytomegalovirus immune evasion. *Curr Top Microbiol Immunol* 2008;**325**:333−59.

286. Lyles DS, Kuzmin I, Rupprecht CE. Rhabdoviridae. In: 6th ed. Knipe DM, Howley PM, editors. *Fields virology*, vol. 1. Philadelphia: Lippincott Williams and Wilkins; 2013. p. 885−922.

Chapter 3

Reverse Vaccinology: Exploiting Genomes for Vaccine Design

E. Del Tordello, R. Rappuoli and I. Delany
GSK Vaccines, Siena, Italy

Reverse vaccinology (RV) defines the process of antigen discovery through the interrogation of an organism's complete antigenic repertoire, as coded in its genomic data. Traditional vaccine development was largely based on Pasteur's principles, which were to "isolate, inactivate, and inject" the disease-causing agent and to translate that process into the production of vaccines that comprised inactivated or live-attenuated microorganisms or purified protein subunits.[1] On the contrary, the RV approach does not require a pathogen to be grown in the laboratory, fostering its application to microorganisms that may not be easily cultivated but at least have an accessible genome sequence.

RV's rise paralleled that of the genomic era at the end of the last century. In 1995 the microbial genome of *Haemophilus influenziae* was sequenced,[2] which paved the way for sequencing genomes of other pathogens. The basic concept of RV—in silico prediction of protective antigens from a genomic sequence—was subsequently proposed in the year 2000 with the identification of novel meningococcal vaccine candidates from the genome sequence of a *Neisseria meningitidis* serogroup B (MenB) strain.[3] This work ultimately led to the licensing of the MenB vaccine (Bexsero) in Europe and the United States, establishing RV as a leading strategy for the rapid and rational development of vaccines against new pathogens or new variants of known pathogens. Over the years, the discipline has evolved, as genomic and bioinformatic methods that were largely responsible for RV's early successes have since been complemented with newer approaches derived from the disciplines of transcriptomics and proteomics. In this chapter, we review past and present applications of RV, trace its technological evolution, and describe the advantages, challenges, and future perspectives for its continued growth within the field of vaccinology.

Human Vaccines: Emerging Technologies in Design and Development.
DOI: http://dx.doi.org/10.1016/B978-0-12-802302-0.00002-9

THE MILESTONE OF THE MenB VACCINE

The first pathogen that RV took on was *N. meningitidis* serogroup B (MenB), a Gram-negative bacterium that causes 50% of meningococcal meningitis cases worldwide[4] (Fig. 3.1). *Neisseria meningitidis* has a polysaccharide capsule that forms the basis for classification into 12 major serogroups, 6 of which are associated with invasive disease (A, B, C, Y, W135, and X). Conjugate vaccines based on capsular polysaccharides induce bactericidal antibodies against all the major serogroups, except for serogroup B. In this case, the capsular polysaccharide is identical to the polysialic acid present in human glycoproteins and is poorly immunogenic. Attempts to identify cross protective vaccine antigens for MenB using traditional approaches were complicated by the variability of surface antigens across different strains.[5] In the late 1990s—because of emerging advancements in gene sequencing—the entire genome sequence of the virulent MenB MC58 strain was determined.[6] Starting from 2158 open reading frames (ORF), bioinformatic analyses identified 570 predicted surface membrane or secreted proteins based on their coding sequence and homology with known virulence factors. Of all candidate

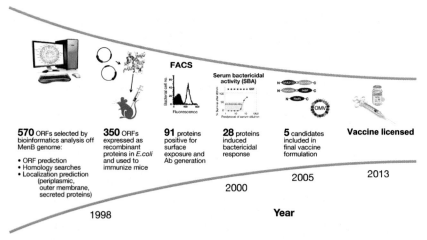

FIGURE 3.1   Reverse vaccinology pipeline applied to MenB. Starting from the 2158 identified open reading frames (ORFs) in the MC58 sequenced genome in 1998, bioinformatic analyses predicted 570 proteins that were either exposed on the surface or secreted or homologous to known virulence factors. Of all the candidate sequences, 350 were successfully cloned in *E. coli*, expressed in soluble form, purified, and used to immunize mice. Immunogenicity and protection were evaluated by testing antisera by flow cytometry and serum bactericidal activity (SBA). Ultimately, 91 of the surface proteins induced antibodies in vivo, of which 28 induced bactericidal antibodies. Five antigens were finally selected based on sequence conservation among a panel of diverse meningococcal strains. They were coformulated with outer membrane vesicles (OMV) and found to be safe, immunogenic and protective studies clinical trials of adults, adolescents and infants, receiving market authorization in 2013.

sequences, 350 were successfully cloned and expressed in *Escherichia coli*. The recombinant proteins were purified, injected into mice and assessed for surface localisation, immunogenicity and protective potential by antisera flow cytometry, serum bactericidal activity (SBA) and animal challenge studies. The screening process resulted in the identification of 91 immunogenic surface proteins, 28 of which elicited bactericidal antibodies.[3] A list of more than two dozen vaccine candidates had been generated within 18 months of sequencing, more than the number identified by all traditional approaches in the preceding 40 years.[7] As a larger number of MenB genomes became available, bacterial genomes from 31 strains worldwide were cross-referenced for antigen conservation. The interrogation of these genomes led to the selection of three conserved, previously unknown bactericidal antigens[8] (Neisseria Heparin Binding Antigen (NHBA), *N. meningitidis* adhesion A (NadA) and factor H binding protein (fHbp)).[9−12] These proteins were formulated together with detergent-extracted outer membrane vesicles from a New Zealand epidemic isolate into a four-component vaccine known as 4CMenB. The vaccine subsequently demonstrated safety and efficacy in more than 7500 infants, children, adolescents and adults[13−15] and received regulatory approval and marketing authorization from the European Medicines Agency in 2013, and from the US Food and Drug Administration in 2015 under the name of Bexsero™.[16]

The RV approach allows for the assessment of all antigens potentially expressed by an organism, without any prior knowledge of their abundance or immunogenicity during the natural history of disease. More importantly, the most protective antigens may not be expressed under in vitro conditions, so that the only way to identify them is to start with an a priori analysis of a pathogen's proteome. Besides identifying novel protective antigens, RV has also led to the discovery of new virulence factors that have advanced our understanding of microbial pathogenesis.[17] The main disadvantage of this approach, however, is that only protein antigens and virulence factors can be identified to the exclusion of polysaccharides, lipopolysaccharides, glycolipids and other CD1-restricted antigens (Table 3.1).

EVOLUTION OF REVERSE VACCINOLOGY OVER 15 YEARS OF APPLICATION

From One Genome to Thousands

The success of the MenB vaccine led, in the following years, to the application of RV to other bacterial pathogens.[18−26] At the same time, the advances in genome sequencing technologies have maintained a rapid pace. As of March 2015, there are, respectively, 3472 and 4601 complete bacterial and viral genomes in the National Center for Biotechnology Information (NCBI) database. Available prokaryotic and viral draft genomes exceed these numbers by more than an order of magnitude. There are also 2400 draft

TABLE 3.1 Comparison Between Conventional and Reverse Vaccinology

	Conventional Vaccinology	Reverse Vaccinology
Antigen identification	Starts with the identification of most abundant antigens during disease	Starts with DNA sequence of the microorganism genome
	Only cultivable microorganisms can be addressed	The microorganism does not need to be cultivated to obtain the genome sequence from different samples
	10–25 antigens are identified by biochemical or genetic tools	Virtually all antigens encoded by the genome are available, based on ORF prediction
Antigen properties	Only highly immunogenic antigens during disease are identified	Antigens even if non-immunogenic during disease can be identified, including non-structural proteins
	Antigens not expressed in vitro cannot be identified	Antigen that are not expressed in vitro or transiently expressed during infection can be identified
	Sequence variability of many of the antigens identified and risk of inducing self immunity	Antigens are selected based on conservation within the circulating strains, and potential self antigens are discarded based on homology with human proteins
	Polysaccharides, lipopplysaccharides, glycolypids, and other CD-1 restricted antigens can be used	Nonproteic antigens cannot be identified

eukaryote genomes, of which 266 are derived from protozoa. The high volume of publically available sequences reflects a trend in falling costs, particularly after 2007 when high-throughput sequencing machines were introduced. Currently, gene sequencing costs approximately $0.10 per megabase pair and no more than $50 for a complete bacterial genome sequence (Fig. 3.2). Moreover, with the availability of different market technologies, the cost of the sequencing equipment has also fallen considerably. As a consequence, most major research centers and clinical microbiology laboratories in high-resource settings house a sequencer that is typically used on a daily basis.

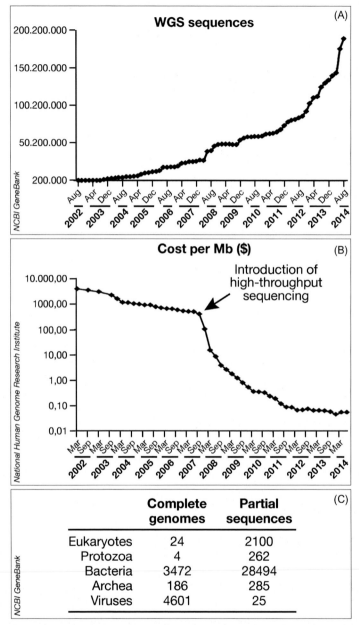

FIGURE 3.2 Genome sequencing evolution in recent years. (A) Number of Whole Genome Shotgun (WSG) sequences available and deposited in NCBI GeneBank from 2002 to 2014. The number has increased over time starting from the first microbial genome in 1995, with exponential growth in recent years. (B) Cost of genome sequencing from 2002 to 2014, indicated as cost per megabase pair (Mb). The cost of sequencing dropped dramatically after 2007, with the introduction of high-throughput sequencing machines. (C). Number of complete and draft genome sequences available up to March 2015 in the NCBI database. *From National Human Research Institute.*

The Pan-Genome and Comparative Genome Analysis

As the field of bioinformatics has matured and multiple genomes from a wide array of bacterial species have become available, it is now possible to compare the whole gene repertoire of multiple isolates of pathogenic and commensal strains of bacteria. These analyses have unexpectedly revealed that bacterial genomes are far more variable than previously thought, particularly when compared to the pathogenicity islands that were once considered to be the major discriminants of a bacterial population.[27] For example, genomic sequences of eight *Streptococcus agalactiae* strains (Group B Streptococcus, GBS) differed from one another in at least 20% of their genes, meaning that there are some genes that are only present in one strain.[24,28] The repertoire of all genes in a set of bacterial genomes sequenced from the same species is termed a "pan-genome"; it comprises a "core-genome" of conserved genes (often associated with essential metabolic functions) and a "dispensable genome" of genes only present in some isolates.[29] The percentages of genes categorized into one group or another differ across bacterial species. The core genome typically represents about 80% of the genome of any given strain, but can fall to as low as 42% in the case of *E. coli*.[30] The dispensable gene pool often includes factors acquired through horizontal transfer between members of the same species or closely related bacteria and represents a key reservoir which bacteria can access to alter their genotype or phenotype as they adapt to changing environmental conditions. Host—pathogen interactions can apply selective pressure that induce these changes. For example, in the setting of pathogen-associated inflammation of the intestinal mucosa, *Salmonella enterica* serovar typhimurium and *E. coli* have been shown to increase their efficiency of plasmids exchange.[31]

Theoretically, the pan-genome of bacteria like GBS is open and unlimited, meaning that, no matter how many strains are interrogated, each genome sequence is likely to uncover new genes.[32] The same is true for *E. coli*.[33] On the contrary, the pan-genome of *Bacillus anthracis* has been entirely described by only four genomes and is therefore considered to be closed.[34] An intermediate model has been proposed for pathogens like *H. influenziae*[35] and *Streptococcus pneumoniae*.[36] In this paradigm, a "supra-genome" is characterized by a finite composite of genes, within species, that defines the complete pan-genome. From the perspective of vaccine discovery and development, antigens selected from the core or dispensable genomes primarily reflect the evolutionary history and lifestyle of each pathogen. While the first impulse may be to look to conserved epitopes from the core genome, antigens from the dispensable genome are under greater selective pressure and may be more likely to elicit protective responses. In the case of GBS, the genomic analysis of eight strains resulted in the development of a vaccine composed of four proteins that, when coformulated, conferred 59—100% protection against a panel of 12 GBS isolates.[24,28] None of these antigens could be classified as universal, because three of them were entirely absent from a fraction of the tested strains. The fourth antigen came from the core genome but was not entirely exposed on the bacterial surface of some strains. The implications are, nonetheless, significant: that comparative genomic analysis employed in RV can deliver broadly protective vaccines, even for microorganisms that have a highly variable genome.

The discovery of dispensable genes has also been instrumental in the design of vaccines against commensal pathogens that occasionally become pathogenic, such as nonpathogenic types of *E. coli*.[25] For uropathogenic strains of *E. coli*, acquisition of a pathogenicity island has resulted in the ability to infect the urinary tract and bloodstream and evade host defenses without compromising the ability to colonize the intestine. Moriel and colleagues compared genome sequences of extra-intestinal pathogenic *E. coli* (ExPEC) to those of nonpathogenic isolates and found 19 genomic islands present only in the former. Nine of the antigens only present in ExPEC were protective in a mouse challenge model. This demonstrated the possibility to develop broadly protective vaccines that do not eliminate the normal flora.[37]

Intra-species genomic diversity suggests a single sequence may not be the representative of the bacterial species as a whole. Moreover, a high level of sequence variability can be observed within core genes and expressed proteins. In the case of *N. meningitidis* fHbp, more than 800 distinct peptide sequences have been identified (http://pubmlst.org/neisseria/fHbp/) and classified into three main groups.[38] *Streptococcus pneumoniae* also has a pilus with structural components—RrgA and RrgB—that vary considerably across strains.[39] Given this heterogeneity, the vaccine candidate selection process has to be streamlined with early systematic analyses of antigen distribution across bacterial populations. This process identifies the main variants that can then inform the design of immunogens that are broadly protective.[40] This technological advance comes with the caveat that sequence conservation of an antigen within a group of bacterial isolates does not necessarily translate into an antigen's ability to confer immunity to all strains. For example, several MenB, GBS, and *E. coli* immunogens that were expected to be cross-protective on the basis of gene sequence conservation failed to protect mice from heterologous bacterial challenges.[3,24,25] One reason for these findings is that the relative abundance of an antigen—conserved or not—on the bacterial surface can vary substantially across strains, due to different levels of expression during infection. Consequently, it is important to complement RV with an assessment of antigens that are expressed in vivo and are more likely to be targeted by antibodies. In many cases antigens that are poorly expressed in vitro can be induced with specific biochemical signals in vivo. As an example, NadA, an adhesin protein and a component of Bexsero is present in approximately 50% of MenB isolates but is expressed variably in vitro, depending on cell growth phase.[41,42] However, it was found to be associated with hypervirulence and was ultimately protective in an infant rat model of bacteremia.[12,43] Downstream analyses demonstrated that NadA expression is highly induced in vivo during experimental bacteremia and by hydroxyphenylacetic acid (HPA) molecular signals, metabolites present in human saliva where MenB is present as a commensal organism.[44]

Advancements in Epidemiology and Data Systems

A fundamental feature of an effective bacterial vaccine is broad coverage within a bacterial population. The availability of complete genome sequences for hundreds of bacterial isolates means that molecular epidemiological data can now inform the initial selection of vaccine candidates. At the advent of the genomic era, bacteria were classified by phenotyping and genotyping methods. The latter was most commonly applied through multilocus sequence typing (MLST).[45] MLST is based on sequencing conserved genes and then defining bacterial sequence types (ST) as allelic profiles. The allele and ST designations group strains into clonal complexes or lineages. However, the variability of housekeeping genes across different bacteria limits the use of MLST to only closely related bacteria. The availability of complete bacterial genomes and so-called whole genome shotgun sequences has revolutionized the way bacterial populations are viewed and classified, particularly from the perspective of vaccine development. As entire sets of genes from each isolate are available, it is possible to assemble genomes, de novo, across diverse isolates.[46,47] In addition to protein-coding genes other components of the genome, such as pseudogenes and intergenic regions, can be considered as typing loci and indexed in the same way. Researchers can apply a set of MLST approaches with different numbers of loci, each suitable for addressing different levels of isolate discrimination. The highest level of resolution, whole-genome MLST, compares all loci within a given isolate to those of other isolates. As few bacteria share all loci, a core genome MLST can still provide high-resolution data across a group of related but not identical isolates.[48]

To establish such a system, it is necessary to store, organize and access genome sequence data in a large but agile database. The new Bacterial Genome Sequence database (BIGSdb) platform applies the MLST approach to whole genome sequencing data and incorporates all the functionality of the software formerly used for the MLST database.[49] BIGSdb links any type of contiguous sequence data, from single genes to complete closed genomes, with provenance and phenotypic data (metadata) for the isolates from which the sequences were originally derived. It also stores allele and locus definitions. Although loci are usually protein-coding genes, any sequence string can be defined as a locus, so that intergenic regions can be included in this approach. Overall, BIGSdb can be considered a population-based annotation tool that enables the identification of particular genes and allelic variants within whole genome sequencing data, maintaining a record of the known variation of that gene across the samples stored in the database.[46]

Another powerful platform that applies genomic analyses to pathogen surveillance and epidemiology is the Denmark-based Center for Genomic Epidemiology (http://www.genomicepidemiology.org). The goal of this project is to provide an open on-line database of rapidly characterized pathogenic and industrial bacteria, even from incomplete genomes. The platform aims to develop statistical and epidemiological tools that integrate genomic data with epidemiologic information. It also allows any laboratory to track the progression of infectious diseases across different geographical regions and environmental niches, so that the genome sequence of a microbe offers access to the genetic diversity that has accumulated in the microbial domain during years of evolution and spread.[50]

Meningococcal Antigen Typing System

Even with advancements in strain classification and data management, accurate predictions of vaccine coverage remain elusive, particularly for multicomponent vaccines where the contribution of more than one antigen must be considered. In the case of meningococcal vaccines, a correlate of protection can be found in the SBA, which determines the ability of immune serum to affect complement-mediated killing of test strains.[51] Due to the diversity in antigen sequences and expression levels, further determinations of effectiveness of the multicomponent MenB (Bexsero) vaccine would require performing SBA against strains collected worldwide, a highly impractical endeavor considering that infants, who are the target population, have limited volumes of serum available for collection. Therefore, the meningococcal antigen typing system (MATS) has been developed to identify MenB strains that have a high likelihood of being covered by Bexsero.[52] The MATS assay combines a series of antigen-specific sandwich ELISA assays, one for each antigen present in the final vaccine formulation, and simultaneously quantifies the amount of these antigens expressed by a given bacterial isolate. By combining the MATS value for each antigen in the vaccine formulation, it is possible to determine whether a specific strain is covered by the vaccine of interest. As a high-throughput assay, it can be used to screen large panels of bacterial strains, making it complementary to genome-based typing and adaptable to protein-based vaccines against other bacteria for which a correlate of protection is known or yet to be identified.

BIOINFORMATICS TOOLS FOR REVERSE VACCINOLOGY

Since the 1991 release of PSORT—a software tool that predicts sites of protein localization in cells[53]—a multitude of bioinformatics tools designed for vaccine discovery have become available. The optimal in silico prediction tool that is used in tandem with an RV-based approach, however, should follow certain principles, including: (1) focus on surface and secreted proteins; (2) interrogate for antigen conservation across different pathogen strains and serotypes; (3) screen for and exclusion of antigens that exhibit molecular mimicry with human proteins; (4) have a preference for antigen sequence homology to proteins associated with virulence or immunogenicity; (5) exclude antigens found in nonpathogenic strains; and (6) focus on antigens that can expressed in a high-throughput manner for vaccine production (e.g., preferentially discard insoluble proteins with multiple transmembrane helices).[54]

Despite the great potential of RV, it can still be challenging to generate a list of promising vaccine candidates. The overall concept of RV—start with a genome and end with a list of vaccine candidates—is relatively straightforward. However, it is not a trivial matter to identify an appropriate bioinformatics tool or database and perform the correct analysis. As the number of available genomes for each pathogen increases, RV is relying more heavily on in silico analyses of large sequence databases. The common strategy now is to link different prediction programs in order to automate the process of high-throughput identification of potential vaccine antigens. Vaxign[55] and NERVE (New Enhanced Reverse Vaccinology Environment)[56] are two examples of vaccine discovery programs being employed for prokaryotes, while Vacceed[57] is dedicated to eukaryotic pathogens. NERVE screens whole bacterial proteomes and integrates multiple analytic algorithms that select antigens based on multiple parameters, including surface-cell localization, adhesion probability, number of transmembrane domains, homology to human proteins, sequence conservation and putative function.[56] Vaxign is a web-based software platform that uses an RV strategy to predict MHC class I and II epitopes.[55] It is available through the Vaccine Investigation and Online Information Network (VIOLIN) and uses a module-based design, where each feature is implemented using an independent program. With a user-friendly interface and integration with other open-source software, this program allows for the selection of features to include in a final vaccine prediction model. Thus far, Vaxign has been used with some success for predicting vaccine targets for *Brucella spp.*,[58] uropathogenic *E. coli*[55] and herpes simplex virus.[59] The last of the commonly used programs, Vacceed, is a collective framework of linked bioinformatics programs, Perl scripts, R functions and Linux shell scripts that work together to initially build a proteome and then model vaccine candidates based on subcellular localization, presence of transmembrane helices and peptide binding to MHC class I molecules. The final output is a ranked list of protein candidates that can then be experimentally validated.[57]

Recently, a new tool has been proposed for the identification of structural and functional features that are known to recur in protective bacterial antigens, a so-called protectome space. This method includes all protective bacterial antigens regardless of their level of protection, mechanism (antibody mediated or cell mediated) or cellular compartmentalization (secreted, surface-associated, and cytoplasmic). When applied to *S. aureus* and GBS, this approach accurately predicted known protective antigens and also identified new candidates.[60] Antigens can also be identified functionally. Adhesins mediate the initial interaction between a pathogen and its cognate host receptor, making them ideal immunogens to include in vaccines.[61] Some important examples include FHA and pertactin for *Bordetella pertussis*[62]; PhtD and PhtE for *S. pneumoniae*[63]; and NadA for *N. meningitidis*.[12] Proteins that play critical roles in pathogenesis can thus serve as both prophylactic and therapeutic targets. The Jenner-Predict server, in particular, facilitates the prediction of protein vaccine candidates based on host−pathogen interactions.[65] It hones in on known functional domains of well-established protein classes, including: adhesins, invasins, porins, flagellins, toxins as well as choline-binding penicillin-binding, transferrin-binding, fibronectin-binding, and solute-binding domains. These tools demonstrate that the collective knowledge on host−pathogen interactions and bacterial pathogenesis enables computer programs to identify vaccine candidates in a rational, mechanistically-rooted manner.[17]

THE USE OF OMICS AS COMPLEMENTARY TOOLS

Functional genomics, in conjunction with genomic sequencing, delivers high-throughput data on gene function and host−pathogen interactions. Transcriptome analyses in the context of different animal or human models, as opposed to in vitro alone, are particularly important for the identification of proteins that are essential for infection, as demonstrated for analyses of *N. meningitidis* or *Salmonella typhi* in ex vivo human blood samples.[66,67] The comparison of commensal and pathogenic strains during infection may also be critical for identifying previously unknown antigens that come from the dispensable genome.[68,69] Next generation RNA-based technologies, such as RNA-seq and tiling microarray can detect protein coding regions, transcriptional units and regulatory elements by analyzing the transcriptome repertoire in an unbiased fashion, resulting in the identification of unpredicted coding sequences, alternative transcripts, and regulatory elements.[70−72] These types of data have increased the accuracy of detecting gene start sites and refined the algorithms for predicting ORFs.

Proteomic technologies also serve as an important complement to the RV approach, as they provide information on the expression, quantity and composition of cell surface proteins.[73] For example, high-throughput mass spectrometry (MS), coupled with two-dimensional gel electrophoresis (2DE) and immunoprecipitation, can quickly and accurately identify proteins that are expressed by the pathogen during infection.[74] Proteomics can also be used to verify predictions offered by genomic analysis. A proteome-derived ORF model for *Mycoplasma pneumoniae*, e.g., confirmed 81% of the predicted ORFs and discovered an additional 16 previously unknown ORFs.[75] In another genome-wide study of *Salmonella typhimurium*, MS-based proteomics confirmed more than 40% of the predicted ORFs, correcting 47 start sites and identifying 12 novel genes not predicted by existing gene-finding algorithms.[76] Proteomics also can be exploited for directly testing the presence and amount of antigens on the surface of bacteria (the so-called surfactome). Rodrıguez-Ortega and colleagues took this approach when they "shaved" the surface of Group A Streptococci (GAS) with mild proteases and scanned the collected peptides with MS to determine the identity and quantity of surface exposed proteins.[77] Gram-negative bacteria have also been examined in a slightly different way: surface antigens are quantified and characterized when membrane vesicles released by wild type bacteria or those genetically modified to weaken the outer membrane stability are run through MS.[78–80]

Immunoproteomics is a branch of proteomic analysis that interrogates the entire antigenic repertoire of a pathogen with the aim of finding antigens that are likely to be immunogenic. In this strategy, 2D-PAGE and Western Blotting or immunoprecipitation are combined with proteomics. The process yields proteins that are bound by sera from a vaccinee or recovered patient.[81–83] Display libraries expressing fragments of a pathogen's proteome can also be screened using serum antibodies of exposed individuals or convalescent patients in order to identify immunogenic antigens expressed during infection (referred to as the "ANTIGENome"). This method has been used to antigenically fingerprint both S. pneumoniae[84] and Streptococcus pyogenes.[85,86]

In the process of developing a vaccine against malaria, investigators encountered many difficulties due to different life stages of the Plasmodium falciparum during infection.[87] In an attempt to solve this problem, Osier and colleagues applied so-called ANTIGENome technology that screened antibody reactivity of sera from a cohort of Kenyan children against a large library of biochemically active merozoite surface and secreted proteins with full-length ectodomains.[88] Antibodies to previously untested or under-studied proteins were found to protect children from clinical malaria with efficacy that was either superior or equivalent to several previously tested vaccine candidates.[89] These findings demonstrated the great potential for a broadly integrated pathway for detecting new immunogens, particularly for complex pathogens. The application of functional genomics to a large panel of pathogen strains has thus proven beneficial, particularly in the context of smaller subsets of genome/strains. The result has been a prioritization of vaccine candidates to be tested in animal models and ultimately advanced to clinical development (Fig. 3.3).[26,90]

RECENT APPLICATIONS TO VACCINES AGAINST BACTERIA, VIRUSES, AND PROTOZOA

Many infectious diseases, particularly those that have caused regional or global outbreaks, are zoonotic in origin.[91,92] Zoonoses tend to jump into human populations with little warning and have high virulence, at least initially, as humans inherently lack immunity. Vaccines have been proposed as one of several interventions that could control the spread of zoonotic infectious diseases and reduce the chance of transmission to human populations. RV approaches have, thus, been applied to the discovery of vaccine candidates against zoonotic pathogens. *Brucella*, the etiologic agent of brucellosis, is a common and widely distributed zoonotic disease. Its high degree of infectiousness and the lack of an approved vaccine for human use make it a viable threat to public health. In order to identify potential vaccine antigens, Gomez and colleagues employed a multistep antigen selection process that used the Vaxign algorithm to predict ORFs that encode outer membrane proteins with antigenic determinants. In the final selection, only five proteins were recombinantly expressed and used for validation, all of which yielded promising immunogenicity data.[58] RV has also been applied to another prototypical zoonosis, *Rickettsia prowazekii*, which is the causative agent of epidemic typhus and is transmitted by the human body louse. Owing to the

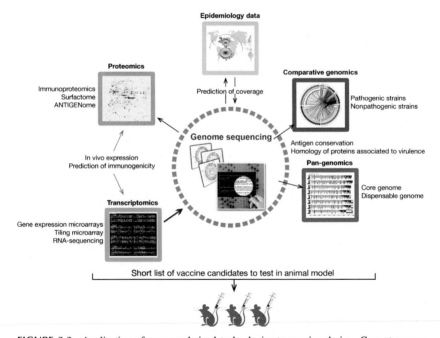

FIGURE 3.3 Application of genome-derived technologies to vaccine design. Current reverse vaccinology approaches start with a comparative analysis of multiple genome sequences in order to identify conserved antigens within a heterogeneous pathogen population or antigens that are present only in pathogenic strains. Epidemiologic data contributes information about the circulating strains for the determination of vaccine coverage. Functional genomics data sets (proteomics, transcriptomics) are incorporated into the selection process, providing information related to the in vivo expression of the selected conserved antigens that cannot be inferred from genomic analysis alone. The integration of these data allow for a fast, cost-effective, ethical, and accurate selection of a short list of candidates.

obligate intracellular lifestyle of rickettsiae, CD8 + T cells are indispensable for protective cellular immunity. Caro-Gomez and colleagues identified and validated four novel *R. prowazekii* vaccine antigen candidates recognized by CD8 + T cells from a set of twelve in silico-defined protein targets[92]. They combined predictions for both proteasome-processing and MHC class-I-binding of the target proteins. Owing to its prior success, RV has also been used for other zoonotic pathogens including *Echinococcus granulosus*[93] and *Francisella tularensis*.[94] In addition to zoonoses, RV has been used for developing veterinary vaccines with the aim of reducing loss of livestock and the associated economic costs. It has recently been applied to the bovine protozoan parasite *Theileria parva*,[95] the swine pathogen *Haemophilus parasuis*[96] and the Gram-negative bacterium *Gallibacterium anatis*, a major cause of salpingitis and peritonitis in commercial poultry.[97] Eukaryotic pathogens prove to be more challenging targets for RV because of their more sophisticated gene structure, antigenic complexity, multiple life-cycle stages, immune evasion strategies and use of intermediate and end host reservoirs.[98] Despite these challenges, the RV pipeline has started to deliver promising results, particularly for leishmaniasis[99] and schistosomiasis.[100]

In the case of viruses, RV provides a way to overcome the problems of pathogen isolation, cultivation and identification. Hepatitis C virus (HCV) is one of the first examples where the viral genome sequence was used to identify putative antigens. The virus is difficult to grow in vitro and the availability of the HCV genome led to the identification of the etiological agent, the recombinant expression of its proteins and the prediction of two envelope proteins (E1 and E2) as possible vaccine antigens.[101] These recombinant proteins have protected chimpanzees from a homologous HCV challenge.[102] Unfortunately, a vaccine against HCV is not yet available due to high variability within circulating strains.[103] A comprehensive and comparative analysis of circulating viral genome sequences is, therefore required to develop a vaccine with broad coverage. Recently, Vaxign software was used to predict vaccine targets for herpesvirus HSV-1,[59] which has also been challenging due to the complexity of the virus's replication cycle and its sophisticated strategies for immune evasion. Using subtractive and pan-genomics approaches, Xiang and colleagues compared ten human herpesviruses genomes to those of 40 non-human herpesviruses to identify seven HSV-1 proteins without orthologues to any other tested nonhuman herpesviruses.[59] Others have employed a similar strategy for human cytomegalovirus (HCMV) where 94 highly conserved membrane-associated or secreted proteins were selected from comparative genome analysis.[104] Selected proteins were expressed, purified and tested for recognition by antibodies in the sera of infected patients. The final screen yielded 36 proteins, including known envelope glycoproteins and antigens that have a role in immune-modulation.[105] An additional ten uncharacterized proteins were selected as well. In the case of highly variable viruses such as HIV and influenza, genomic information may be exploited to design entirely unconventional vaccine targets that could include nonstructural proteins.[106,107] In the case of influenza, however, a solution could come from the identification of conserved sequences within the viral genome. A number of investigators have focused on the highly conserved stalk region of the hemagglutinin surface protein of influenza, including Steel and colleagues who successfully used an RV approach to identify immunogens that elicited antibodies that were cross-protective in a murine influenza model.[108]

CHALLENGES AND FUTURE PERSPECTIVES FOR REVERSE VACCINOLOGY

The first analysis of the *N. meningitidis* genome has paved the way for a generation of vaccines to be discovered via in silico methods. Currently, RV approaches start with a comparative analysis of multiple genome sequences in order to identify conserved antigens within a heterogeneous pathogen population. Genomics, transcriptomics, proteomics and other -OMICS data sets can now be integrated into the selection process and provide information on cellular localization and in vivo expression that cannot be inferred from genomic analysis alone (Fig. 3.3). These data, combined with other information gained from flow cytometry and immunoproteomics, enable a rapid and discriminating selection of candidates. The end result is an immunogen selection process that is more cost-effective and ethical, reducing the need for animal experiments.[90]

As the cost of sequencing has fallen dramatically, a significant barrier has been overcome to utilizing high-throughput functional genomics with greater frequency. The primary bottleneck for RV now is the availability of bioinformatics tools that are able to seamlessly integrate genomic, proteomic and epidemiologic data for the prediction of immunogenic antigens. Still, there are an increasing number of bioinformatics tools becoming available that Filippini et al. have collectively termed "functional informatics."[54] The development of novel tools for RV will help address some of the remaining questions about the accessibility of surface antigens, antigen masking and protein degradation and posttranslational modification of proteins, particularly for eukaryotic pathogens.[54] Currently, gene finder programs are not able to consistently predict the exon−intron structures of eukaryotic genes or account for alternative splicing. In the context of viruses, one of the main limitations of RV is the inability to predict protein complexes or expression levels.[104] However, ribosome profiling technology has expanded the range of polypeptides produced beyond previously annotated ORFs, suggesting that the effective coding potential of viral genomes is higher than predicted.[109]

As the importance of cellular immunity to vaccine efficacy has become increasingly recognized, it is likely that RV will delve into this area by capitalizing on the growing field of immunomics.[110] Genomic information can be used to scan the entire repertoire of CD4 + and CD8 + T cell epitopes.

Measuring and predicting cellular immunity is particularly important in cases where T cell responses are relevant for protection and clearance of infection (or establishment of a chronic infection if the response is impaired) as for many viral and bacterial infections (e.g., HIV, HCV, TB, malaria). Although technically challenging, in recent years the development of specific bioinformatic tools for CD4 + and CD8 + T cell epitopes [111–113] have been instrumental to elucidating the breadth of potential antigens, particularly for complex pathogens like mycobacteria and plasmodia.[114,115]

The RV approach is not per se applicable to already well-defined vaccine antigens that are too variable or unstable to induce protective immune response. Improvements in X-ray crystallography, nuclear magnetic resonance imaging and electron microscopy, however, yielded accurate structural information of major vaccine antigens that can be used for modifications that make them better immunogens.[116] This approach, termed structural vaccinology, is complimenting RV antigen selection strategies. RV has demonstrated to be a fast and comprehensive tool for antigen discovery and is often the first approach used in the challenge to identify vaccine candidates for emerging pathogens.

ACKNOWLEDGMENTS

We thank Giorgio Corsi for the artwork.

REFERENCES

1. Plotkin SA. Vaccines: the fourth century. *Clin Vaccine Immunol* 2009;**16**:1709–19.
2. Fleischmann RD, Adams MD, White O, et al. Whole-genome random sequencing and assembly of *Haemophilus influenzae* Rd. *Science* 1995;**269**:496–512.
3. Pizza M, Scarlato V, Masignani V, et al. Identification of vaccine candidates against serogroup B meningococcus by whole-genome sequencing. *Science* 2000;**287**:1816–20.
4. Stephens DS, Greenwood B, Brandtzaeg P. Epidemic meningitis, meningococcaemia, and *Neisseria meningitidis*. *Lancet* 2007;**369**:2196–210.
5. Stephens DS. Biology and pathogenesis of the evolutionarily successful, obligate human bacterium *Neisseria meningitidis*. *Vaccine* 2009;**27**(Suppl. 2):B71–7.
6. Tettelin H, Saunders NJ, Heidelberg J, et al. Complete genome sequence of *Neisseria meningitidis* serogroup B strain MC58. *Science* 2000;**287**:1809–15.
7. Rappuoli R. Reverse vaccinology, a genome-based approach to vaccine development. *Vaccine* 2001;**19**:2688–91.
8. Giuliani MM, Adu-Bobie J, Comanducci M, et al. A universal vaccine for serogroup B meningococcus. *Proc Natl Acad Sci USA* 2006;**103**:10834–9.
9. Serruto D, Spadafina T, Ciucchi L, et al. *Neisseria meningitidis* GNA2132, a heparin-binding protein that induces protective immunity in humans. *Proc Natl Acad Sci USA* 2010;**107**:3770–5.
10. Seib KL, Scarselli M, Comanducci M, Toneatto D, Masignani V. *Neisseria meningitidis* factor H-binding protein fHbp: a key virulence factor and vaccine antigen. *Expert Rev Vaccines* 2015;**14**:841–59.

11. Madico G, Welsch JA, Lewis LA, et al. The meningococcal vaccine candidate GNA1870 binds the complement regulatory protein factor H and enhances serum resistance. *J Immunol* 2006;**177**:501−10.

12. Capecchi B, Adu-Bobie J, Di Marcello F, et al. *Neisseria meningitidis* NadA is a new invasin which promotes bacterial adhesion to and penetration into human epithelial cells. *Mol Microbiol* 2005;**55**:687−98.

13. Toneatto D, Ismaili S, Ypma E, Vienken K, Oster P, Dull P. The first use of an investigational multicomponent meningococcal serogroup B vaccine (4CMenB) in humans. *Hum Vaccin* 2011;**7**:646−53.

14. Santolaya ME, O'Ryan ML, Valenzuela MT, et al. Immunogenicity and tolerability of a multicomponent meningococcal serogroup B (4CMenB) vaccine in healthy adolescents in Chile: a phase 2b/3 randomised, observer-blind, placebo-controlled study. *Lancet* 2012;**379**:617−24.

15. Findlow J, Borrow R, Snape MD, et al. Multicenter, open-label, randomized phase II controlled trial of an investigational recombinant Meningococcal serogroup B vaccine with and without outer membrane vesicles, administered in infancy. *Clin Infect Dis* 2010;**51**:1127−37.

16. Martin NG, Snape MD. A multicomponent serogroup B meningococcal vaccine is licensed for use in Europe: what do we know, and what are we yet to learn? *Expert Rev Vaccines* 2013;**12**:837−58.

17. Delany I, Rappuoli R, Seib KL. Vaccines, reverse vaccinology, and bacterial pathogenesis. *Cold Spring Harb Perspect Med* 2013;**3**:a012476.

18. Wizemann TM, Heinrichs JH, Adamou JE, et al. Use of a whole genome approach to identify vaccine molecules affording protection against *Streptococcus pneumoniae* infection. *Infect Immun* 2001;**69**:1593−8.

19. Ross BC, Czajkowski L, Hocking D, et al. Identification of vaccine candidate antigens from a genomic analysis of *Porphyromonas gingivalis*. *Vaccine* 2001;**19**:4135−42.

20. Montigiani S, Falugi F, Scarselli M, et al. Genomic approach for analysis of surface proteins in *Chlamydia pneumoniae*. *Infect Immun* 2002;**70**:368−79.

21. Ariel N, Zvi A, Grosfeld H, et al. Search for potential vaccine candidate open reading frames in the *Bacillus anthracis* virulence plasmid pXO1: in silico and in vitro screening. *Infect Immun* 2002;**70**:6817−27.

22. Betts JC. Transcriptomics and proteomics: tools for the identification of novel drug targets and vaccine candidates for tuberculosis. *IUBMB Life* 2002;**53**:239−42.

23. Etz H, Minh DB, Henics T, et al. Identification of in vivo expressed vaccine candidate antigens from *Staphylococcus aureus*. *Proc Natl Acad Sci USA* 2002;**99**:6573−8.

24. Maione D, Margarit I, Rinaudo CD, et al. Identification of a universal Group B Streptococcus vaccine by multiple genome screen. *Science* 2005;**309**:148−50.

25. Moriel DG, Bertoldi I, Spagnuolo A, et al. Identification of protective and broadly conserved vaccine antigens from the genome of extraintestinal pathogenic *Escherichia coli*. *Proc Natl Acad Sci USA* 2010;**107**:9072−7.

26. Bagnoli F, Fontana MR, Soldaini E, et al. Vaccine composition formulated with a novel TLR7-dependent adjuvant induces high and broad protection against *Staphylococcus aureus*. *Proc Natl Acad Sci USA* 2015;**112**:3680−5.

27. Hacker J, Kaper JB. Pathogenicity islands and the evolution of microbes. *Annu Rev Microbiol* 2000;**54**:641−79.

28. Tettelin H, Medini D, Donati C, Masignani V. Towards a universal group B Streptococcus vaccine using multistrain genome analysis. *Expert Rev Vaccines* 2006;**5**:687−94.

29. Tettelin H, Riley D, Cattuto C, Medini D. Comparative genomics: the bacterial pangenome. *Curr Opin Microbiol* 2008;**11**:472−7.

30. Touchon M, Hoede C, Tenaillon O, et al. Organised genome dynamics in the *Escherichia coli* species results in highly diverse adaptive paths. *PLoS Genet* 2009;**5**:e1000344.

31. Stecher B, Denzler R, Maier L, et al. Gut inflammation can boost horizontal gene transfer between pathogenic and commensal Enterobacteriaceae. *Proc Natl Acad Sci USA* 2012;**109**:1269−74.

32. Tettelin H, Masignani V, Cieslewicz MJ, et al. Genome analysis of multiple pathogenic isolates of *Streptococcus agalactiae*: implications for the microbial "pan-genome". *Proc Natl Acad Sci USA* 2005;**102**:13950−5.

33. Rasko DA, Rosovitz MJ, Myers GS, et al. The pangenome structure of *Escherichia coli*: comparative genomic analysis of *E. coli* commensal and pathogenic isolates. *J Bacteriol* 2008;**190**:6881−93.

34. Medini D, Donati C, Tettelin H, Masignani V, Rappuoli R. The microbial pan-genome. *Curr Opin Genet Dev* 2005;**15**:589−94.

35. Hogg JS, Hu FZ, Janto B, et al. Characterization and modeling of the Haemophilus influenzae core and supragenomes based on the complete genomic sequences of Rd and 12 clinical nontypeable strains. *Genome Biol* 2007;**8**:R103.

36. Hiller NL, Janto B, Hogg JS, et al. Comparative genomic analyses of seventeen *Streptococcus pneumoniae* strains: insights into the pneumococcal supragenome. *J Bacteriol* 2007;**189**:8186−95.

37. Moriel DG, Rosini R, Seib KL, Serino L, Pizza M, Rappuoli R. *Escherichia coli*: great diversity around a common core. *mBio*. 2012;3.

38. Masignani V, Comanducci M, Giuliani MM, et al. Vaccination against *Neisseria meningitidis* using three variants of the lipoprotein GNA1870. *J Exp Med* 2003;**197**:789−99.

39. Muzzi A, Moschioni M, Covacci A, Rappuoli R, Donati C. Pilus operon evolution in *Streptococcus pneumoniae* is driven by positive selection and recombination. *PLoS One* 2008;**3**:e3660.

40. Scarselli M, Arico B, Brunelli B, et al. Rational design of a meningococcal antigen inducing broad protective immunity. *Sci Transl Med* 2011;**3**:91ra62.

41. Martin P, van de Ven T, Mouchel N, Jeffries AC, Hood DW, Moxon ER. Experimentally revised repertoire of putative contingency loci in *Neisseria meningitidis* strain MC58: evidence for a novel mechanism of phase variation. *Mol Microbiol* 2003;**50**:245−57.

42. Comanducci M, Bambini S, Brunelli B, et al. NadA, a novel vaccine candidate of *Neisseria meningitidis*. *J Exp Med* 2002;**195**:1445−54.

43. Litt DJ, Savino S, Beddek A, et al. Putative vaccine antigens from *Neisseria meningitidis* recognized by serum antibodies of young children convalescing after meningococcal disease. *J Infect Dis* 2004;**190**:1488−97.

44. Metruccio MM, Pigozzi E, Roncarati D, et al. A novel phase variation mechanism in the meningococcus driven by a ligand-responsive repressor and differential spacing of distal promoter elements. *PLoS Pathog* 2009;**5**:e1000710.

45. Maiden MC, Bygraves JA, Feil E, et al. Multilocus sequence typing: a portable approach to the identification of clones within populations of pathogenic microorganisms. *Proc Natl Acad Sci USA* 1998;**95**:3140−5.

46. Jolley KA, Maiden MC. Automated extraction of typing information for bacterial pathogens from whole genome sequence data: *Neisseria meningitidis* as an exemplar. *Eurosurveillance* 2013;**18**:20379.

47. Sheppard SK, Jolley KA, Maiden MC. A gene-by-gene approach to bacterial population genomics: whole genome MLST of campylobacter. *Genes* 2012;**3**:261−77.

48. Maiden MC, Jansen van Rensburg MJ, Bray JE, et al. MLST revisited: the gene-by-gene approach to bacterial genomics. *Nat Rev Microbiol* 2013;**11**:728–36.
49. Jolley KA, Maiden MC. BIGSdb: scalable analysis of bacterial genome variation at the population level. *BMC Bioinformatics* 2010;**11**:595.
50. Ciccarelli FD, Doerks T, von Mering C, Creevey CJ, Snel B, Bork P. Toward automatic reconstruction of a highly resolved tree of life. *Science* 2006;**311**:1283–7.
51. Borrow R, Balmer P, Miller E. Meningococcal surrogates of protection − serum bactericidal antibody activity. *Vaccine* 2005;**23**:2222–7.
52. Donnelly J, Medini D, Boccadifuoco G, et al. Qualitative and quantitative assessment of meningococcal antigens to evaluate the potential strain coverage of protein-based vaccines. *Proc Natl Acad Sci USA* 2010;**107**:19490–5.
53. Nakai K, Kanehisa M. Expert system for predicting protein localization sites in gram-negative bacteria. *Proteins* 1991;**11**:95–110.
54. Vivona S, Gardy JL, Ramachandran S, et al. Computer-aided biotechnology: from immuno-informatics to reverse vaccinology. *Trends Biotechnol* 2008;**26**:190–200.
55. He Y, Xiang Z, Mobley HL. Vaxign: the first web-based vaccine design program for reverse vaccinology and applications for vaccine development. *J Biomed Biotechnol* 2010;**2010**:297505.
56. Vivona S, Bernante F, Filippini F. NERVE: new enhanced reverse vaccinology environment. *BMC Biotechnol* 2006;**6**:35.
57. Goodswen SJ, Kennedy PJ, Ellis JT. Vacceed: a high-throughput in silico vaccine candidate discovery pipeline for eukaryotic pathogens based on reverse vaccinology. *Bioinformatics* 2014;**30**:2381–3.
58. Gomez G, Pei J, Mwangi W, Adams LG, Rice-Ficht A, Ficht TA. Immunogenic and invasive properties of *Brucella melitensis* 16M outer membrane protein vaccine candidates identified via a reverse vaccinology approach. *PLoS One* 2013;**8**:e59751.
59. Xiang Z, He Y. Genome-wide prediction of vaccine targets for human herpes simplex viruses using Vaxign reverse vaccinology. *BMC Bioinformatics* 2013;**14**(Suppl. 4):S2.
60. Altindis E, Cozzi R, Di Palo B, et al. Protectome analysis: a new selective bioinformatics tool for bacterial vaccine candidate discovery. *Mol Cell Proteomics* 2015;**14**:418–29.
61. Gamez G, Hammerschmidt S. Combat pneumococcal infections: adhesins as candidates for protein-based vaccine development. *Curr Drug Targets* 2012;**13**:323–37.
62. Brennan MJ, Shahin RD. Pertussis antigens that abrogate bacterial adherence and elicit immunity. *Am J Respir Crit Care Med* 1996;**154**:S145–9.
63. Khan MN, Pichichero ME. Vaccine candidates PhtD and PhtE of *Streptococcus pneumoniae* are adhesins that elicit functional antibodies in humans. *Vaccine* 2012;**30**:2900–7.
64. Jaiswal V, Chanumolu SK, Gupta A, Chauhan RS, Rout C. Jenner-Predict server: prediction of protein vaccine candidates (PVCs) in bacteria based on host-pathogen interactions. *BMC Bioinformatics* 2013;**14**:211.
65. Echenique-Rivera H, Muzzi A, Del Tordello E, et al. Transcriptome analysis of *Neisseria meningitidis* in human whole blood and mutagenesis studies identify virulence factors involved in blood survival. *PLoS Pathog* 2011;**7**:e1002027.
66. Sheikh A, Charles RC, Sharmeen N, et al. In vivo expression of *Salmonella enterica* serotype Typhi genes in the blood of patients with typhoid fever in Bangladesh. *PLoS Negl Trop Dis* 2011;**5**:e1419.
67. Grifantini R, Bartolini E, Muzzi A, et al. Gene expression profile in *Neisseria meningitidis* and *Neisseria lactamica* upon host-cell contact: from basic research to vaccine development. *Ann NY Acad Sci* 2002;**975**:202–16.

68. Grifantini R, Bartolini E, Muzzi A, et al. Previously unrecognized vaccine candidates against group B meningococcus identified by DNA microarrays. *Nat Biotechnol* 2002;**20**:914−21.

69. Mader U, Nicolas P, Richard H, Bessieres P, Aymerich S. Comprehensive identification and quantification of microbial transcriptomes by genome-wide unbiased methods. *Curr Opin Biotechnol* 2011;**22**:32−41.

70. Toledo-Arana A, Dussurget O, Nikitas G, et al. The Listeria transcriptional landscape from saprophytism to virulence. *Nature* 2009;**459**:950−6.

71. Sharma CM, Hoffmann S, Darfeuille F, et al. The primary transcriptome of the major human pathogen *Helicobacter pylori*. *Nature* 2010;**464**:250−5.

72. Grandi G. Antibacterial vaccine design using genomics and proteomics. *Trends Biotechnol* 2001;**19**:181−8.

73. Walters MS, Mobley HL. Bacterial proteomics and identification of potential vaccine targets. *Expert Rev Proteomics* 2010;**7**:181−4.

74. Jaffe JD, Berg HC, Church GM. Proteogenomic mapping as a complementary method to perform genome annotation. *Proteomics* 2004;**4**:59−77.

75. Ansong C, Tolic N, Purvine SO, et al. Experimental annotation of post-translational features and translated coding regions in the pathogen *Salmonella typhimurium*. *BMC Genomics* 2011;**12**:433.

76. Rodriguez-Ortega MJ, Norais N, Bensi G, et al. Characterization and identification of vaccine candidate proteins through analysis of the group A Streptococcus surface proteome. *Nat Biotechnol* 2006;**24**:191−7.

77. Vaughan TE, Skipp PJ, O'Connor CD, et al. Proteomic analysis of *Neisseria lactamica* and *Neisseria meningitidis* outer membrane vesicle vaccine antigens. *Vaccine* 2006;**24**:5277−93.

78. Jang KS, Sweredoski MJ, Graham RL, Hess S, Clemons Jr. WM. Comprehensive proteomic profiling of outer membrane vesicles from *Campylobacter jejuni*. *J Proteomics* 2014;**98**:90−8.

79. Berlanda Scorza F, Doro F, Rodriguez-Ortega MJ, et al. Proteomics characterization of outer membrane vesicles from the extraintestinal pathogenic *Escherichia coli* DeltatolR IHE3034 mutant. *Mol Cell Proteomics* 2008;**7**:473−85.

80. Roy K, Bartels S, Qadri F, Fleckenstein JM. Enterotoxigenic *Escherichia coli* elicits immune responses to multiple surface proteins. *Infect Immun* 2010;**78**:3027−35.

81. Falisse-Poirrier N, Ruelle V, ElMoualij B, et al. Advances in immunoproteomics for serological characterization of microbial antigens. *J Microbiol Methods* 2006;**67**:593−6.

82. Christodoulides M. Neisseria proteomics for antigen discovery and vaccine development. *Expert Rev Proteomics* 2014;**11**:573−91.

83. Giefing C, Meinke AL, Hanner M, et al. Discovery of a novel class of highly conserved vaccine antigens using genomic scale antigenic fingerprinting of pneumococcus with human antibodies. *J Exp Med* 2008;**205**:117−31.

84. Fritzer A, Senn BM, Minh DB, et al. Novel conserved group A streptococcal proteins identified by the antigenome technology as vaccine candidates for a non-M protein-based vaccine. *Infect Immun* 2010;**78**:4051−67.

85. Deng J, Bi L, Zhou L, et al. *Mycobacterium tuberculosis* proteome microarray for global studies of protein function and immunogenicity. *Cell Rep* 2014;**9**:2317−29.

86. Doolan DL, Apte SH, Proietti C. Genome-based vaccine design: the promise for malaria and other infectious diseases. *Int J Parasitol* 2014;**44**:901−13.

87. Osier FH, Mackinnon MJ, Crosnier C, et al. New antigens for a multicomponent blood-stage malaria vaccine. *Sci Transl Med* 2014;**6**:247ra102.

88. Osier FH, Fegan G, Polley SD, et al. Breadth and magnitude of antibody responses to multiple *Plasmodium falciparum* merozoite antigens are associated with protection from clinical malaria. *Infect Immun* 2008;**76**:2240−8.

89. Bensi G, Mora M, Tuscano G, et al. Multi high-throughput approach for highly selective identification of vaccine candidates: the Group A Streptococcus case. *Mol Cell Proteomics* 2012;**11**. M111.015693.

90. Keeling MJ, Gilligan CA. Bubonic plague: a metapopulation model of a zoonosis. *Proc Biol Sci* 2000;**267**:2219−30.

91. Hald T, Vose D, Wegener HC, Koupeev T. A Bayesian approach to quantify the contribution of animal-food sources to human salmonellosis. *Risk Anal* 2004;**24**:255−69.

92. Caro-Gomez E, Gazi M, Goez Y, Valbuena G. Discovery of novel cross-protective *Rickettsia prowazekii* T-cell antigens using a combined reverse vaccinology and in vivo screening approach. *Vaccine* 2014;**32**:4968−76.

93. Gan W, Zhao G, Xu H, et al. Reverse vaccinology approach identify an *Echinococcus granulosus* tegumental membrane protein enolase as vaccine candidate. *Parasitol Res* 2010;**106**:873−82.

94. Chandler JC, Sutherland MD, Harton MR, et al. *Francisella tularensis* LVS surface and membrane proteins as targets of effective post-exposure immunization for tularemia. *J Proteome Res* 2015;**14**:664−75.

95. Graham SP, Honda Y, Pelle R, et al. A novel strategy for the identification of antigens that are recognised by bovine MHC class I restricted cytotoxic T cells in a protozoan infection using reverse vaccinology. *Immunome Res* 2007;**3**:2.

96. Hong M, Ahn J, Yoo S, et al. Identification of novel immunogenic proteins in pathogenic *Haemophilus parasuis* based on genome sequence analysis. *Vet Microbiol* 2011;**148**:89−92.

97. Bager RJ, Kudirkiene E, da Piedade I, et al. In silico prediction of *Gallibacterium anatis* pan-immunogens. *Vet Res* 2014;**45**:80.

98. Mutapi F, Billingsley PF, Secor WE. Infection and treatment immunizations for successful parasite vaccines. *Trends Parasitol* 2013;**29**:135−41.

99. John L, John GJ, Kholia T. A reverse vaccinology approach for the identification of potential vaccine candidates from Leishmania spp. *Appl Biochem Biotechnol* 2012;**167**:1340−50.

100. de Oliveira Lopes D, de Oliveira FM, do Vale Coelho IE, et al. Identification of a vaccine against schistosomiasis using bioinformatics and molecular modeling tools. *Infect Genet Evol* 2013;**20**:83−95.

101. Reed KD, Meece JK, Henkel JS, Shukla SK. Birds, migration and emerging zoonoses: West Nile virus, lyme disease, influenza A and enteropathogens. *Clin Med Res* 2003;**1**:5−12.

102. Choo QL, Kuo G, Ralston R, et al. Vaccination of chimpanzees against infection by the hepatitis C virus. *Proc Natl Acad Sci USA* 1994;**91**:1294−8.

103. Drummer HE. Challenges to the development of vaccines to hepatitis C virus that elicit neutralizing antibodies. *Front Microbiol* 2014;**5**:329.

104. Bruno L, Cortese M, Rappuoli R, Merola M. Lessons from reverse vaccinology for viral vaccine design. *Curr Opin Virol* 2015;**11**:89−97.

105. Fouts AE, Chan P, Stephan JP, Vandlen R, Feierbach B. Antibodies against the gH/gL/UL128/UL130/UL131 complex comprise the majority of the anti-cytomegalovirus (anti-CMV) neutralizing antibody response in CMV hyperimmune globulin. *J Virol* 2012;**86**:7444−7.

106. Kwong PD, Mascola JR, Nabel GJ. Rational design of vaccines to elicit broadly neutralizing antibodies to HIV-1. *Cold Spring Harb Perspect Med* 2011;**1**:a007278.

107. Cassone A, Rappuoli R. Universal vaccines: shifting to one for many. *mBio* 2010;1.

108. Steel J, Lowen AC, Wang TT, et al. Influenza virus vaccine based on the conserved hemagglutinin stalk domain. *mBio* 2010;1.

109. Ingolia NT. Ribosome profiling: new views of translation, from single codons to genome scale. *Nat Rev Genet* 2014;**15**:205–13.

110. Sette A, Rappuoli R. Reverse vaccinology: developing vaccines in the era of genomics. *Immunity* 2010;**33**:530–41.

111. Nielsen M, Lund O, Buus S, Lundegaard C. MHC class II epitope predictive algorithms. *Immunology* 2010;**130**:319–28.

112. Zhang Q, Wang P, Kim Y, et al. Immune epitope database analysis resource (IEDB-AR). *Nucleic Acids Res* 2008;**36**:W513–18.

113. Lin HH, Ray S, Tongchusak S, Reinherz EL, Brusic V. Evaluation of MHC class I peptide binding prediction servers: applications for vaccine research. *BMC Immunol* 2008;**9**:8.

114. Blythe MJ, Zhang Q, Vaughan K, et al. An analysis of the epitope knowledge related to mycobacteria. *Immunome Res* 2007;**3**:10.

115. Vaughan K, Blythe M, Greenbaum J, et al. Meta-analysis of immune epitope data for all plasmodia: overview and applications for malarial immunobiology and vaccine-related issues. *Parasite Immunol* 2009;**31**:78–97.

116. Dormitzer PR, Grandi G, Rappuoli R. Structural vaccinology starts to deliver. *Nat Rev Microbiol* 2012;**10**:807–13.

Chapter 4

Virus-Like Particle and Nanoparticle Vaccines

M. Kanekiyo[1] and C.B. Buck[2]
[1]*Vaccine Research Center, NIAID, National Institutes of Health, Bethesda, MD, United States,*
[2]*Center for Cancer Research, NCI, National Institutes of Health, Bethesda, MD, United States*

INTRODUCTION

Currently licensed vaccines can be divided into three broad categories: (1) genetically attenuated "live" pathogens that remain replication-competent but have greatly diminished ability to cause disease; (2) "killed" pathogens that have been chemically inactivated; and (3) isolated "subunit" fragments of pathogens. The first two categories are represented, respectively, by the classic oral (Sabin) and injectable (Salk) poliovirus vaccines. During their initial development, it was quickly appreciated that the live-attenuated immunogen confers durable immunity against wild-type poliovirus replication in vaccinated individuals (i. e., sterilizing immunity). In contrast, the inactivated immunogen generally provides more transient protection and primarily serves to prevent the spread of poliovirus to the central nervous system, as opposed to fully preventing viral replication in the gut. These patterns are recapitulated in the responses elicited by other vaccines. For example, live-attenuated immunogens, such as measles and smallpox vaccines, provide long-term sterilizing immunity, while killed pathogen vaccines induce more transient responses that require periodic boosting.[1] The differences can be at least partially attributed to the fact that live immunogens display a variety of pathogen-associated molecular patterns (PAMPs) that engage innate antimicrobial sensors, such as toll-like receptors (TLRs).[2] This contrasts with replication-incompetent immunogens, which lack these innate "danger" signals and therefore induce a diminished, delayed, and less durable immune response.

Subunit vaccine responses tend to follow the same pattern as killed pathogen vaccines. A familiar example is the tetanus toxoid vaccine, which requires periodic boosting to maintain protective levels of tetanus toxin-neutralizing

Human Vaccines: Emerging Technologies in Design and Development.
DOI: http://dx.doi.org/10.1016/B978-0-12-802302-0.00003-0

antibodies. In the current review, we focus on a new class of more immunogenic subunit vaccines in which the immunogen of interest is organized into a multivalent array that resembles the surface of geometrically rigid virions. The resulting immunogens, termed "virus-like particles" (VLPs), are typically composed of recombinant virion structural proteins that self-assemble into nanoparticles in the absence of viral genomic DNA or RNA. It is now well established that properly assembled VLPs can induce potent, diverse, and durable serum antibody responses that are comparable to responses against live or live-attenuated pathogens. The remarkable potency of rigidly multivalent subunit immunogens has been most comprehensively documented in studies of current commercial VLP-based vaccines against human papillomaviruses (HPVs).[3,4] An emerging view is that at least some types of VLP immunogens, including current HPV vaccines, fall into a special class of subunit vaccine that can show the same potency and durability as live-attenuated immunogens. Recent clinical trials have demonstrated that VLP immunogens can even be potent enough to overcome the self-tolerance of human B cells, allowing the induction of auto-antibody responses of therapeutic interest.[5,6]

Not all VLP antigens show the same high immunogenicity as HPV vaccines. For example, the commercial hepatitis B virus (HBV) vaccine, which is comprised of VLPs assembled from the HBV surface (S) envelope protein, induces relatively poor antibody titers that decline over time.[7] It may be that the S protein is arrayed in a relatively mobile and flexible way and thus fails to qualify as a geometrically rigid multivalent structure. Similar flexibility issues might explain why emerging VLP-based vaccines against Dengue virus appear not to have elicited stable high-titer neutralizing antibody responses in clinical trials.[8]

HUMORAL RECOGNITION OF VIRUSES

Nearly all known animal viruses have virion diameters in the 10–1000 nanometer (nm) range. Smaller (<500 nm) virions can passively traffic through lymphatic system and can also be directly taken up by immune cells such as macrophages, dendritic cells, and B cells. Either pathway efficiently brings antigens to the lymph nodes, where adaptive immune responses can be induced. In the setting of the lymph node, successfully transported virions are taken up by specialized macrophages in the subcapsular sinus of the draining lymph node. Virions are then transferred to follicular dendritic cells (FDCs) where they are directly presented to B cells. Durable attachment to FDCs can be enhanced by decoration of the presented antigen with low affinity IgM antibodies or complement components.[9] When antigen-specific surface immunoglobulins (Igs) on the B cell (B cell receptors (BCRs)) recognize the antigen, these BCRs form microclusters to promote a signaling cascade that activates the B cell. The recognized antigen can then be endocytosed and processed for presentation on an MHC class II protein, which in turn recruits the help of antigen-specific CD4 + T cells.

RIGIDLY MULTIVALENT IMMUNOGENS: THEORY AND PRACTICE

In 1993, Bachmann, Zinkernagel and colleagues showed that B cells recognize multivalent antigens with repetitive 50−100 angstrom (Å) spacing in a distinctive way that leads to potent induction of cell activation and survival signals.[10] Rigid epitope spacing of this type is commonly found on the surface of many types of virions but is rare among vertebrate self antigens. In fact, some of the few host protein complexes with 50−100 Å spacing are immune gene products, such as IgM antibodies, complement component C1q, and collectins like the mannose binding lectin. Repetitive spacing can thus be seen as a type of PAMP that B cells have evolved to specifically detect via engagement of cell surface BCRs. Strong B cell responses can be elicited by other types of PAMP signals through engagement of Toll-like receptors (TLRs) or by persistent interaction with FDCs through IgM or C1q. However, the Bachmann-Zinkernagel effect operates independently of conventional adjuvant signaling. Instead, epitope spacing and rigidity appear to be the primary variable in triggering this effect.[11] There is some indirect evidence that multivalent immunogens trigger a special type of signaling separate from adjuvant effects. This comes from the observation that it is extremely difficult or perhaps impossible to generate hybridomas from mice immunized with rigid virus-like particles under dosing schedules typically used for production of monoclonal antibodies.[12,4,13]

Using mouse model systems, Übelhart and colleagues have recently proposed a model in which soluble monovalent antigens trigger signaling primarily through IgM-isotype BCRs, while multivalent antigens are able to trigger signaling through IgD-isotype BCRs found on fully mature B cells.[14] The hinge region of each surface Ig isotype is critical for determining sensitivity to rigidly multivalent antigens. A current hypothesis is that internalization of multivalent antigens via IgD may lead to enhanced presentation of the antigen to CD4 + T cells.[15]

Initially, it was unclear whether the Bachmann-Zinkernagel effect would be applicable to humans. The extraordinary success of the current rigid multivalent VLP vaccines against HPV has confirmed its relevance to human populations. Participants in early trials of HPV vaccines who received only one dose of the vaccine demonstrated high titer neutralizing antibody responses that plateaued for at least six years after vaccination (Fig. 4.1).[16,17] Booster doses of the HPV vaccine cause only incremental increases in antibody titers. This type of response stands in dramatic contrast to more conventional immunogens, such as traditional tetanus toxoid vaccines, where booster doses trigger major, albeit temporary, rises in neutralizing antibody titers (Fig. 4.2).[18] A possible interpretation is that a given B cell's initial contact with the VLP immunogen triggers a differentiation pathway—presumably mediated by IgD BCRs—that predisposes the cell to expand and differentiate into a set of

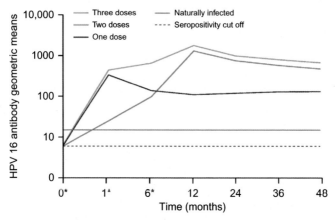

FIGURE 4.1 Serological responses to an HPV VLP vaccine.

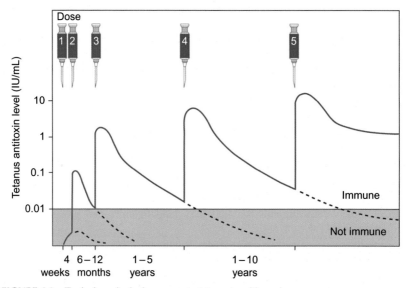

FIGURE 4.2 Typical serological response to tetanus toxoid vaccine.

long-lived plasma cells that reside in the bone marrow without necessarily passing through a durable memory B cell phenotype.

NATURALLY ICOSAHEDRAL VIRIONS

The success of current HPV vaccines demonstrates that recombinant particles assembled from naturally rigid icosahedral virion proteins can provide durable antibody-based sterilizing immunity to pathogenic viruses. A surprising feature of HPV vaccines is that they induce antibody responses capable of cross-protecting women against infection with HPV serotypes that aren't present in the vaccine preparation.[19] A newer version of the HPV vaccine contains VLPs that represent nine different HPV serotypes, and the presence of multiple antigens in the single vaccine has little impact on the induction of responses to all nine types.

The outcome of HPV VLP vaccines suggests a promising path for developing VLP vaccines for other diverse families of viruses with naturally rigid icosahedral virions. The knobby nonenveloped icosahedral surface of polyomavirus virions is one example. Polyomaviruses are so similar to papillomavirus virions that the two viral families were originally classified into a single viral family, the *Papovaviridae*, based on their appearance in electron micrographs. VLPs based on two pathogenic human polyomaviruses known as BKV and JCV are currently under investigation as possible vaccine immunogens.[20–22] In a "compassionate use" case study, an elderly immunodeficient patient given an experimental JCV VLP vaccine demonstrated a remarkably high JCV-neutralizing serological titer of approximately 25 million. The result is consistent with the idea that polyomavirus VLP immunogens may be at least as potent as current HPV VLP vaccines.

A number of other important human pathogens have naturally rigid icosahedral surfaces. One example is Chikungunya virus, a member of the *Alphavirus* family. VLPs assembled from the icosahedrally rigid envelope glycoprotein of Chikungunya virus have elicited high-titer neutralizing antibody responses in both animal models and in human trials.[23,24] Noroviruses represent another promising target for VLP vaccine development. Results from clinical trials of VLP-based vaccines against norovirus are currently under consideration by the US Food and Drug Administration. The recent success of a VLP-based vaccine against canine parvovirus suggests that comparable VLP-based vaccines against human parvovirus B19 should be feasible.

Human rhinoviruses are naturally icosahedral non-enveloped viruses and thus may represent another facile target for VLP vaccine development. Rhinoviruses collectively cause 70% of mild upper respiratory infections in humans. Although there are at least 100 known rhinovirus serotypes, it may eventually be possible to construct a panel of recombinant rhinovirus VLPs for inclusion of a multi-VLP vaccine analogous to the nine-serotype HPV VLP vaccine. Based on the assumption that a multi-VLP rhinovirus vaccine immunogen would, like HPV VLP vaccines, elicit at least some degree of cross-neutralization of rhinovirus serotypes not contained in the vaccine, this approach could theoretically offer broad protection against the common cold. The project could serve to pave the way for the development of VLP-based vaccines against viruses in the Picornaviridae family, including emerging pathogens such as EV68, which has been associated with flaccid paralysis.

As mentioned above, VLPs based on flaviviruses, such as dengue virus, have so far elicited poor immunogenicity despite the potentially icosahedral display of the surface pre-membrane (prM) and envelope (E) proteins. Structural studies of dengue virions and VLPs indicate that E can exist in a range of highly distinct conformations. A major conformational shift is triggered by proteolysis of the PrM by the cellular protease furin. Structure-guided design and engineering of more complete proteolysis of recombinant dengue VLPs might result in more rigid display of a uniformly "mature" herringbone configuration of E proteins, thereby more effectively triggering the Backmann-Zinkernagel effect. The initial work that revealed the Bachmann-Zinkernagel effect relied on use of a vesicular stomatitis virus (VSV) model system. Like other members of the viral family *Rhabdoviridae*, the surface envelope glycoprotein (G) of VSV is not icosahedrally ordered. VSV G is, however, arrayed at very high density on the bullet-shaped surface of the virion. This suggests that strict geometric rigidity is not necessarily required to trigger the Bachmann-Zinkernagel effect and that other forms of extremely high-density polyvalency can suffice.

SYNTHETIC STRUCTURE-BASED NANOPARTICLE PLATFORMS

Advances in structural biology and nanotechnology have opened new opportunities for the design of synthetic vaccine immunogens on the basis of atomic-level information. Designs mimic a number of biological macromolecules including cargo proteins, multimeric enzymes, subviral particles, viral capsids, and other self-assembling proteins. Typically, vaccine antigens are displayed on these scaffolding molecules to form defined nanostructures such as nanoparticles, nanotubes and nanosheets. Vaccine antigens are typically conjugated to these scaffolds by genetic fusion either (i.e., single polypeptide construct), through adaptor molecules (e.g., streptavidin-biotin interactions) or through covalent chemical crosslinking. Each approach has advantages and challenges, and the best approach may vary depending on the target immunogen. Genetic fusion is not always feasible as many fusion partners disrupt the assembly of the underlying multimeric scaffold protein. On the other hand, genetic fusion systems allow precise control over antigen orientation and occupancy (i.e., surface density of the antigen) and can be generated with simple production pipelines. Genetic fusion systems have recently been used to create self-assembling vaccine immunogens for the influenza virus[25,26], HIV-1,[27] respiratory syncytial virus (RSV),[28] and Epstein-Barr virus (EBV).[29] In the influenza nanoparticle studies, the viral hemagglutinin (HA) envelope protein or truncated HA stem protein was able to trimerize at the three fold symmetric axes of a self-assembled nanoparticle based on a bacterial ferritin protein. Many other types of viral envelope proteins exist as homotrimers on the surface of natural virions. Examples of viruses with trimeric envelope proteins include HIV-1, RSV, human metapneumovirus, coronaviruses (e.g., Middle Eastern respiratory syndrome virus) and Ebola viruses. Thus, the suitability of the ferritin platform for rigid multivalent display of trimeric antigens opens opportunities to create complex nanoparticulate vaccine immunogens. It is also possible to use other symmetric axes of ferritin or encapsulin, which is another bacterial protein that has recently been successfully engineered as a nanoparticle vaccine platform.[29]

Viral Capsid Scaffolds

Viral capsids were the first and now the most widely used nanoparticle scaffolds for displaying antigens of interest in a rigid multivalent array. In one of its earliest uses in 1987, VLPs assembled from the core protein of hepatitis B virus (HBcAg) were able to display an exogenous foot-and-mouse disease virus (FMDV) epitope.[30] The ~27 nm HBcAg particles were able to elicit FMDV-specific immune responses in animals at a substantially higher magnitude compared to responses elicited by a nonnanoparticulate β-galactosidase scaffold or free peptide epitope alone. Since then, as structural biology and biochemical techniques have continued to mature, other viral capsids and proteins have been utilized to display various epitopes and protein antigens.[6] One advantage of using viral capsids, such as HBcAg or bacteriophage-derived capsid proteins, is that the VLP can be produced in high-yield bacterial expression systems that are easily scalable for vaccine manufacturing. Typically, the extension of genes or insertion of exogenous target antigen is limited in these platforms by either size, shape, orientation of the antigen, or a combination of these factors. Thus, it is often difficult to display larger antigens, such an entire viral envelope protein. For example, the HBcAg is a versatile platform to present some relatively large proteins but proper nanoparticle assembly is disrupted if the N- and C-termini of the antigen of interest are too distant from one another. This problem has been partially resolved by introducing enzymatic cleavage sites near the HBcAg-insertion site, thereby releasing one terminus of the insert and relaxing the core protein scaffold to allow particle assembly.[31]

In prokaryotic expression systems it is possible to incorporate unnatural amino acids into nanoscaffolds, making them suitable for chemical conjugation. Multiple VLP systems have used this technology to conjugate exogenous antigens on to the surface of particles. The method is especially powerful if the antigen of interest requires a specific tertiary or quaternary structure, disulfide bond formation or glycosylation or other posttranslational modifications to elicit the desired immune response. Conjugation of the antigen to an acceptor scaffold allows separate expression of the scaffold and the antigen in heterologous expression and purification systems. The efficiency of chemical conjugation varies for different systems as the distribution, occupancy and orientation of the antigen on the scaffold surface can be difficult to control. These factors can be partly manipulated by conjugation conditions (i.e., concentration of antigen and scaffold) or genetic design (restricting the number of reactive residues on both scaffold and antigen). Recently, an alternative conjugation technique has been described on the P22 bacteriophage capsid system, in which an adaptor protein called Dec (decoration protein) is used to link the target antigen to the particle scaffold.[32] The Dec protein assembles into trimers so that it can, in principle, be attached to trimeric proteins such as influenza HA, HIV-1 envelope, Ebola virus glycoprotein, RSV fusion protein or coronavirus spike proteins. Another recent study reports use of the *Streptococcus pyogenes* fibronectin binding protein-based SpyTag/SpyCatcher system for predictable covalent linkage of antigens.[33] One of the earliest but now well-established systems made use of chemical conjugation of biotin to an HPV VLP scaffold surface, thereby allowing tetrameric streptavidin to serve as a "bridge" to display a biotinylated protein antigen.[11]

Self-Assembling Proteinaceous Nanoparticles

In addition to virion structural proteins, there are many groups of proteins that naturally form higher-order multimers that are geometrically rigid and suitable for vaccine antigen display. Some of these multivalent nonviral proteins are chaperones or enzyme complexes that require a multimeric state for specific biological functions. Ferritin is perhaps the best-characterized example of a nonviral protein nanoparticle that has been engineered for multiple applications, including semiconductors, in vivo contrast agents and diagnostic biosensors. It has also been used as a carrier protein to deliver therapeutic agents and vaccine antigens. Early attempts primarily focused on attaching simple peptide epitopes to the surface of self-assembled ferritin particles using tractable prokaryotic production systems. As outlined above, the ferritin platform has shown robust humoral immunogenicity in animal models and seems likely to move forward toward to clinical trials.

Another successful example in this category is based on a bacterial enzyme, lumazine synthase. Analogous to ferritin, a single subunit of this protein self-assembles into an icosahedral particle ($T = 1$), with 60 identical building blocks, thus having potential use for multivalent display of monomeric antigens.[27] Although ferritin and lumazine synthase nanoparticles are relatively small in diameter ($\sim 12-20$ nm) compared to typical virions or viral capsids, some recombinant antigen-decorated nanoparticles in this size range have now been shown to recapitulate the Bachmann-Zinkernagel effect. Furthermore, it has been demonstrated that certain mutations in lumazine synthase can lead to assembly of larger nanoparticles.[34]

In a study of EBV gp350-nanoparticle vaccine candidates, the receptor-binding domain of EBV gp350 was linked either to ferritin or to another slightly larger (24 nm) diameter scaffold assembled from a bacterial encapsulin protein subunit. Both types of antigen-nanoparticles elicited similar magnitudes of humoral response to the EBV antigen, suggesting that nanoparticle size did not significantly affect immunogenicity in this context.[29]

The encapsulin platform has also been engineered to encapsidate proteins in the lumen of the nanoparticle by attaching a specific signal sequence on the encapsidated proteins.[35] This accentuates the potential for creating nanoparticulate vaccine immunogens that deliver encapsidated adjuvant molecules, such as co-stimulatory molecules or TLR agonists. These proteinaceous nanoparticles can be made in mammalian cells by simply introducing a secretion signal sequence. The secreted subunit protein (and fused antigen) can spontaneously self-assemble into nanoparticles in the milieu of the ER lumen and be purified as nanoparticles from culture supernatant by straightforward chromatography techniques. An advantage of this approach is that the fused antigen of interest can fold properly and acquire a natural pattern of post-translational modifications such as glycosylation, which is known to be critical for proper folding of many viral envelope proteins. Many additional classes of nanoparticles remain to be explored as vaccine antigen display scaffolds. Some examples of unexplored areas in this discipline include bacterial microcompartment complexes as scaffolds[36] and vertebrate immune system components that recognize multivalent antigens. The latter may include complement component C1q, IgM, mannose binding protein (MBP) or related highly oligomeric lectins. These vertebrate-derived scaffolds might have the advantage of persisting on FDCs or other immune cells that have specific receptors for C1q, IgM, or MBP.

A next generation of nanoparticles could include features such as conditional assembly/disassembly or higher order and regulated coassembly. Prototype systems for conditional assembly have been explored with an engineered ferritin with a redesigned monomer-monomer interface carrying metal-binding site that "smoothens" the surface and renders assembly dependent on the presence of the metal ions.[37] At present, there are no examples of using proteinaceous nanoparticles to accommodate multiple inserts, which might allow display of hetero-oligomeric antigens of interest. It is possible that this type of display could be achieved using scaffolds that are comprised of more than one type of building block. Such platforms might include a two-subunit insect ferritin[38] or a three-subunit F420-reducing hydrogenese nanoparticle.[39] Alternatively, it might be possible to obtain the same complexity with "split" designs by breaking down a single subunit protein into two or more smaller parts. In sum, the field of vaccine design utilizing the synthetic proteinaceous self-assembled nanoparticle platforms is already well past its infancy and a few of the aforementioned candidates will soon be entering human clinical trials. It is likely that this new class of immunogens will possesses superior immunogenicity and will provide for rapid, flexible and scalable manufacturing of subunit vaccines in the near future.

De Novo Design of Synthetic Self-Assembling Nanoparticles

Modern computational approaches are increasingly poised to solve challenging structural biology questions that have previously been impervious to experimental investigation. The first attempts to utilize synthetic building blocks to make a self-assembling molecule as a scaffold to display exogenous antigens started with very simple structures—two helices linked with a loop—to recreate two-, three- and fivefold symmetry axes of canonical icosahedral particles.[40] As protein modeling has become increasingly accurate and reliable, larger and more complex subunit building blocks are being designed. Such protein building blocks can now be designed in silico to self-assemble into a quaternary complexes, such as nanoparticles.[41,42] These computational approaches might offer a path to implementing functions such as conditional assembly/disassembly or may offer improved immunogenicity for more challenging antigens, such as the structurally plastic HIV-1 Env protein.

CONCLUSION

VLPs and self-assembling proteinaceous nanoparticles are powerful platforms to present antigens to the humoral immune system. These platforms represent a geometrically rigid repetitive array of antigens that, in contrast to soluble monomeric protein subunits, are capable of robustly triggering PAMP-mediated immune stimulation of B cells. In addition to the highly successful current VLP-based vaccines against HPVs, many other VLP/nanoparticle-based vaccine candidates have recently entered preclinical and clinical trials. The potential applications of this new class of vaccine platforms are very broad and seem poised to serve as an important next generation of vaccines.

REFERENCES

1. Amanna IJ, Carlson NE, Slifka MK. Duration of humoral immunity to common viral and vaccine antigens. *N Engl J Med* 2007;**357**:1903—15. Available from: http://dx.doi.org/10.1056/NEJMoa066092.
2. Maisonneuve C, Bertholet S, Philpott DJ, De Gregorio E. Unleashing the potential of NOD- and toll-like agonists as vaccine adjuvants. *Proc Natl Acad Sci USA* 2014;**111**:12294—9. Available from: http://dx.doi.org/10.1073/pnas.1400478111.
3. Schiller JT, Lowy DR. Understanding and learning from the success of prophylactic human papillomavirus vaccines. *Nat Rev Microbiol* 2012;**10**:681—92. Available from: http://dx.doi.org/10.1038/nrmicro2872.
4. Schiller JT, Lowy DR. Raising expectations for subunit vaccine. *J Infect Dis* 2015;**211**:1373—5. Available from: http://dx.doi.org/10.1093/infdis/jiu648.
5. Chackerian B, Frietze KM. Moving towards a new class of vaccines for non-infectious chronic diseases. *Expert Rev Vaccines* 2016;**15**:561—3. Available from: http://dx.doi.org/10.1586/14760584.2016.1159136.
6. Frietze KM, Peabody DS, Chackerian B. Engineering virus-like particles as vaccine platforms. *Curr Opin Virol* 2016;**18**:44—9. Available from: http://dx.doi.org/10.1016/j.coviro.2016.03.001.
7. Leuridan E, Van Damme P. Hepatitis B and the need for a booster dose. *Clin Infect Dis* 2011;**53**:68—75. Available from: http://dx.doi.org/10.1093/cid/cir270.

8. Goo L, Pierson TC. Dengue virus: bumps in the road to therapeutic antibodies. *Nature* 2015;**524**:295−6. Available from: http://dx.doi.org/10.1038/524295a.

9. Link A, et al. Innate immunity mediates follicular transport of particulate but not soluble protein antigen. *J Immunol* 2012;**188**:3724−33. Available from: http://dx.doi.org/10.4049/jimmunol.1103312.

10. Bachmann MF, et al. The influence of antigen organization on B cell responsiveness. *Science* 1993;**262**:1448−51.

11. Chackerian B, Lenz P, Lowy DR, Schiller JT. Determinants of autoantibody induction by conjugated papillomavirus virus-like particles. *J Immunol* 2002;**169**:6120−6.

12. Pastrana DV, Pumphrey KA, Cuburu N, Schowalter RM, Buck CB. Characterization of monoclonal antibodies specific for the Merkel cell polyomavirus capsid. *Virology* 2010;**405**:20−5. Available from: http://dx.doi.org/10.1016/j.virol.2010.06.022.

13. Bachmann MF, Jennings GT. Vaccine delivery: a matter of size, geometry, kinetics and molecular patterns. *Nat Rev Immunol* 2010;**10**:787−96. Available from: http://dx.doi.org/10.1038/nri2868.

14. Ubelhart R, et al. Responsiveness of B cells is regulated by the hinge region of IgD. *Nat Immunol* 2015;**16**:534−43. Available from: http://dx.doi.org/10.1038/ni.3141.

15. Kim YM, et al. Monovalent ligation of the B cell receptor induces receptor activation but fails to promote antigen presentation. *Proc Natl Acad Sci USA* 2006;**103**:3327−32. Available from: http://dx.doi.org/10.1073/pnas.0511315103.

16. Schiller JT, Muller M. Next generation prophylactic human papillomavirus vaccines. *Lancet Oncol* 2015;**16**:e217−25. Available from: http://dx.doi.org/10.1016/S1470-2045(14)71179-9.

17. Kreimer AR, et al. Efficacy of fewer than three doses of an HPV-16/18 AS04-adjuvanted vaccine: combined analysis of data from the Costa Rica Vaccine and PATRICIA trials. *Lancet Oncol* 2015;**16**:775−86. Available from: http://dx.doi.org/10.1016/S1470-2045(15)00047-9.

18. Roper MH, Vandelaer JH, Gasse FL. Maternal and neonatal tetanus. *Lancet* 2007;**370**:1947−59. Available from: http://dx.doi.org/10.1016/S0140-6736(07)61261-6.

19. Draper E, et al. A randomized, observer-blinded immunogenicity trial of Cervarix and Gardasil Human Papillomavirus vaccines in 12−15 year old girls. *PLoS One* 2013;**8**: e61825. Available from: http://dx.doi.org/10.1371/journal.pone.0061825.

20. Pastrana DV, et al. Neutralization serotyping of BK polyomavirus infection in kidney transplant recipients. *PLoS Pathog* 2012;**8**:e1002650. Available from: http://dx.doi.org/10.1371/journal.ppat.1002650.

21. Pastrana DV, et al. BK polyomavirus genotypes represent distinct serotypes with distinct entry tropism. *J Virol* 2013;**87**:10105−13. Available from: http://dx.doi.org/10.1128/JVI.01189-13.

22. Ray U, et al. JC polyomavirus mutants escape antibody-mediated neutralization. *Sci Transl Med* 2015;**7**:306ra151. Available from: http://dx.doi.org/10.1126/scitranslmed.aab1720.

23. Akahata W, et al. *Nature Medicine* 2010;**16**:334−8.

24. Chen LJ, et al. *Lancet* 2014;**384**:2046−52.

25. Kanekiyo M, et al. Self-assembling influenza nanoparticle vaccines elicit broadly neutralizing H1N1 antibodies. *Nature* 2013;**499**:102−6. Available from: http://dx.doi.org/10.1038/nature12202.

26. Yassine HM, et al. Hemagglutinin-stem nanoparticles generate heterosubtypic influenza protection. *Nat Med* 2015;**21**:1065−70. Available from: http://dx.doi.org/10.1038/nm.3927.

27. Jardine J, et al. Rational HIV immunogen design to target specific germline B cell receptors. *Science* 2013;**340**:711−16. Available from: http://dx.doi.org/10.1126/science.1234150.

28. Schickli JH, et al. Palivizumab epitope-displaying virus-like particles protect rodents from RSV challenge. *Eur J Clin Investig* 2015;**125**:1637−47. Available from: http://dx.doi.org/10.1172/JCI78450.

29. Kanekiyo M, et al. Rational design of an epstein-barr virus vaccine targeting the receptor-binding site. *Cell* 2015;**162**:1090−100. Available from: http://dx.doi.org/10.1016/j.cell.2015.07.043.

30. Clarke BE, et al. Improved immunogenicity of a peptide epitope after fusion to hepatitis B core protein. *Nature* 1987;**330**:381−4. Available from: http://dx.doi.org/10.1038/330381a0.

31. Walker A, Skamel C, Vorreiter J, Nassal M. Internal core protein cleavage leaves the hepatitis B virus capsid intact and enhances its capacity for surface display of heterologous whole chain proteins. *J Biol Chem* 2008;**283**:33508−15. Available from: http://dx.doi.org/10.1074/jbc.M805211200.

32. Schwarz B, et al. Symmetry controlled, genetic presentation of bioactive proteins on the P22 virus-like particle using an external decoration protein. *ACS Nano* 2015. Available from: http://dx.doi.org/10.1021/acsnano.5b03360.

33. Brune KD, et al. Plug-and-display: decoration of virus-like particles via isopeptide bonds for modular immunization. *Sci Rep* 2016;**6**:19234. Available from: http://dx.doi.org/10.1038/srep19234.

34. Zhang X, et al. Multiple assembly states of lumazine synthase: a model relating catalytic function and molecular assembly. *J Mol Biol* 2006;**362**:753−70. Available from: http://dx.doi.org/10.1016/j.jmb.2006.07.037.

35. Rurup WF, Snijder J, Koay MS, Heck AJ, Cornelissen JJ. Self-sorting of foreign proteins in a bacterial nanocompartment. *J Am Chem Soc* 2014;**136**:3828−32. Available from: http://dx.doi.org/10.1021/ja410891c.

36. Kerfeld CA, Heinhorst S, Cannon GC. Bacterial microcompartments. *Annu Rev Microbiol* 2010;**64**:391−408. Available from: http://dx.doi.org/10.1146/annurev.micro.112408.134211.

37. Huard DJ, Kane KM, Tezcan FA. Re-engineering protein interfaces yields copper-inducible ferritin cage assembly. *Nat Chem Biol* 2013;**9**:169−76. Available from: http://dx.doi.org/10.1038/nchembio.1163.

38. Hamburger AE, West Jr. AP, Hamburger ZA, Hamburger P, Bjorkman PJ. Crystal structure of a secreted insect ferritin reveals a symmetrical arrangement of heavy and light chains. *J Mol Biol* 2005;**349**:558−69. Available from: http://dx.doi.org/10.1016/j.jmb.2005.03.074.

39. Vitt S, et al. The F(4)(2)(0)-reducing [NiFe]-hydrogenase complex from *Methanothermobacter marburgensis*, the first X-ray structure of a group 3 family member. *J Mol Biol* 2014;**426**:2813−26. Available from: http://dx.doi.org/10.1016/j.jmb.2014.05.024.

40. Raman S, Machaidze G, Lustig A, Aebi U, Burkhard P. Structure-based design of peptides that self-assemble into regular polyhedral nanoparticles. *Nanomedicine* 2006;**2**:95−102. Available from: http://dx.doi.org/10.1016/j.nano.2006.04.007.

41. King NP, et al. Computational design of self-assembling protein nanomaterials with atomic level accuracy. *Science* 2012;**336**:1171−4. Available from: http://dx.doi.org/10.1126/science.1219364.

42. King NP, et al. Accurate design of co-assembling multi-component protein nanomaterials. *Nature* 2014;**510**:103−8. Available from: http://dx.doi.org/10.1038/nature13404.

Part III

Immune Monitoring

Chapter 5

Systems Vaccinology

M. Rolland[1,2] and M.A. Eller[1,2]

[1]*US Military HIV Research Program, Walter Reed Army Institute of Research, Silver Spring, MD, United States*, [2]*The Henry M. Jackson Foundation for the Advancement of Military Medicine, Inc., Bethesda, MD, United States*

Effective vaccines for numerous pathogens—including malaria, tuberculosis (TB), and human immunodeficiency virus (HIV)—remain elusive despite decades of research. Scores of HIV vaccine strategies have been proposed, with more than 550 phase I trials registered at clinicaltrials.gov (April 24, 2016). However, just six phase IIb/III vaccine efficacy trials have been conducted, testing only four concepts. The main challenge for pathogens like HIV or TB is the lack of a straightforward pathway for advanced development because of the absence of a robust correlate of protection. Such a correlate of immunity that associates with the incidence of infection is crucial to guide the development of vaccines, as it provides a way to down-select vaccine candidates that fail to induce the desired immune response. As such, correlates of protection serve as the fundamental "go/no-go" criterion to advance candidates through early stages of development. Current strategies to better define vaccine correlates of immunity are moving beyond the standard characterization of cellular and humoral responses to also analyze host and microbial genetic parameters using systematic OMICS-guided approaches. These novel strategies harness the power of "big data" for the purpose of identifying vaccine candidates that offer the best chance of providing protective immunity.

DEFINITION

Systems vaccinology, a term coined by Bali Pulendran in 2010,[1] studies the complex interactions underlying vaccine-induced immunity in humans by integrating multiple types of data (e.g., serology, genomics transcriptomics, proteomics, metabolomics), primarily through the use of mathematical and computational modeling. By analyzing the large data sets that are generated

Human Vaccines: Emerging Technologies in Design and Development.
DOI: http://dx.doi.org/10.1016/B978-0-12-802302-0.00004-2

by high-throughput technologies, these systematic methods seek an in-depth, integrated understanding of the molecular networks mediating vaccine immunity. This general approach is also used to identify the key molecular signatures that are induced early after vaccination. Specifically, the goal is to identify specific signals that predict: (1) the safety profile of a vaccine candidate; (2) the quality of the vaccine-induced immune response as measured by magnitude, breadth, functionality, and duration; and (3) the vaccine efficacy. Such signatures may help to elucidate the mechanisms by which vaccines mediate protection, predict safety and efficacy outcomes of candidate vaccines, and therefore, provide surrogate endpoints for vaccine trials.

QUESTIONS TO ADDRESS

While the ultimate goal of systems vaccinology is to find immune correlates predictive of vaccine-mediated protection, this strategy is also meant to elucidate the interactions between pathogen and host immunity. There are several key questions that, if addressed within this framework, can facilitate vaccine development. It is critical to understand what components of a microbial antigen, the adjuvant and the platform for presentation that make up the vaccine are responsible for the elicited immune response and how these components interact with one another. An understanding of their contributions will better inform decisions on vaccine delivery routes, immunization schedules and boosting strategies. Systems analyses have already shown that vaccine-mediated immunity and protection differ according to antigen class (polysaccharide vs conjugate[2]) and general platform (live-attenuated vs inactivated), all in the context of various pathogens.[3,4]

The granular elucidation of vaccine-induced immunity requires a detailed and panoramic characterization of the affinity, breadth, functionality, magnitude and specificity of neutralizing and nonneutralizing antibody responses as well as the antigen specificity, breadth, magnitude, polyfunctionality, and Th1/Th2-skewing influences of the T cell response. While these parameters are typical measurements in standard assays, the added value of systems vaccinology is to evaluate them in the context of a multifactorial analysis. Such studies may help discern if specific vaccines, and their components, bias toward humoral or cellular immunity, thereby revealing areas of synergy and antagonism to be, respectively, maximized and avoided.

A systems -based approach toward understanding vaccine immunity also requires a comprehensive framework to analyze innate immunity and its interaction with adaptive immunity. By systematically parsing out the contributions of the two arms of immunity, vaccine regimens can be optimized so as to potentiate the earliest innate and adaptive immune responses.[5] Early engagement of innate effectors, acceleration of the peak adaptive responses and earlier establishment memory responses would likely then provide a pathway toward vaccine candidates with more durable immunity.

In the search for clear and reproducible surrogates of vaccine-induced immunity, it is clear that efforts must focus on those markers that are present in the peripheral blood, as mucosal tissue and lymph node specimens, though desirable, are often inaccessible for analysis in clinical trials. In addition to vaccine trials, natural infection cohort studies play an important role in providing a window into the markers that are associated with or confer immunity or recovery in the convalescent survivors of a particular disease. Animal models can help compliment human studies by providing easier access to tissue samples. As future human studies are designed, however, innovative strategies will need to be developed to make determination of tissue-specific immunity a more feasible endeavor.

METHODS

In recent years, remarkable advances in high-throughput analytic platforms such as transcriptomics, metabolomics, and genomics, have made large-scale correlative analyses possible.

Transcriptomics

Transcriptomics is arguably the most widespread and reliable high-throughput technology in use in the growing discipline of systems vaccinology. It accurately quantifies the expression of all gene transcripts in individual cells or cell populations. Transcriptome analysis also provides information about regulatory elements—such as splice junctions, exon usage, or transcription initiation sites—and the sequences of human leukocyte antigen (HLA) alleles or T cell and B cell receptor molecules, all of which dictate the potency, breadth, and durability of the adaptive immune response. The power of vaccine transcriptomics was first demonstrated in a study by Querec and colleagues in a study of the response to the yellow fever vaccine, YF-17D.[6] They showed that gene signatures derived from the transcriptional profiling of peripheral blood mononuclear cells performed in the first week following vaccination were predictive of YF-17D immunogenicity. Briefly, a gene signature that included complement protein C1qβ and eukaryotic translation initiation factor 2α kinase 4 predicted strong CD8 + T cell responses, while a signature that included the B cell growth factor TNFRS17 was predictive of the magnitude of the neutralizing antibody response. The peak change for most genes occurred on day 7 postvaccination. However, other studies showed changes earlier after vaccination. For example, Bucasas and colleagues showed that a gene expression signature that included 494 genes, measured within 24 hours of vaccination correlated with the magnitude of the neutralizing antibody response against influenza.[3,7] Subsequent analyses of other vaccine responses have added support to the utility of analyzing transcriptome profiles as a means to understanding the molecular changes that make for a robust vaccine response.

Systems Serology

Although neutralizing antibody titers have been the cornerstone for defining a vaccine immune response, some vaccine studies have demonstrated protection in the absence of an association with antibody levels.[8-12] These findings, primarily in the areas of HIV and Dengue vaccine development, have paved the way for investigations of the nonneutralizing Fc-mediated functions of antibodies. Chung and colleagues, for example, recently described a comprehensive computational approach, named "systems serology," to analyze the multifaceted humoral responses elicited in four HIV vaccine-trials.[4] They showed that each vaccine elicited a unique Fc-profile that corresponded to a specific humoral response pattern. This systems serology approach, which comprises an integrated suite of assays linking antibody structural features to effector functions, could also be valuable to dissect the humoral responses induced by vaccines against other pathogens.

High-throughput methods in the context of systems serology assess the determinants of antigen recognition and downstream functional consequences. Investigators first define the key biophysical properties of the antibodies: isotype, subclass, and Fc receptor usage. These features are then linked to an analysis of effector functions, that include antibody dependent -cellular cytotoxicity (ADCC), -cellular phagocytosis (ADCP), -complement deposition (ADCD), -neutrophil activation (ADNA), and -viral inhibition (ADVI). This approach holds promise for providing insights into how a vaccine can afford protection without the need for high levels of neutralizing antibodies.

Cellular Characterization

Flow cytometry is the primary technology used to define cell populations and their functions[13,14] and the capabilities for cell-discrimination have increased rapidly (17-color options are currently widespread[15]). Large populations of heterogeneous cells and the diversity of phenotype and function make it challenging to identify signatures of protection (Fig. 5.1A). Future advances will likely rely on the integration of several different parameters: (1) single cell phenotypes; (2) combinatorial technologies; and (3) novel computational analytic methods. Single cell technologies will become more powerful as flow cytometric platforms are multiplexed so as to tease out specificities of intertwined immune responses (Fig. 5.1B). Conventional flow cytometry is limited by the availability of reagents and the complexities of spectral overlap. A newer approach, mass cytometry or cytometry time of flight (CyTOF), labels antibodies with isotopes of rare-earth metals,[17] resulting in minimal spectral overlap and a theoretical capacity to distinguish up to 100 unique characteristics simultaneously.[18] For example, in one study, investigators used 36 metal-tagged cellular markers to assess the functionality and phenotype of CD8 + T cells; finding marked diversity within the "central memory" compartment

(A)

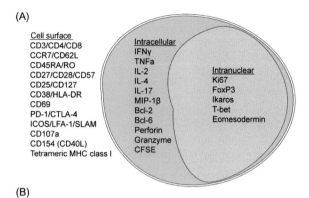

(B)

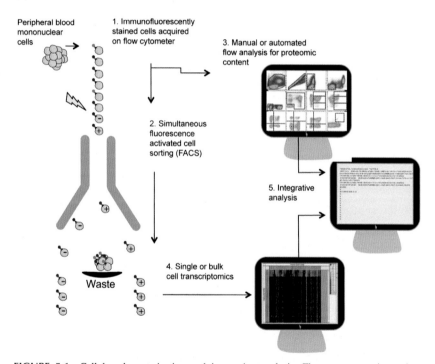

FIGURE 5.1 Cellular characterization and integrative analysis. Flow cytometry is used to determine the magnitude, breadth, phenotype, and polyfunctionality of cells following vaccination. (A) Phenotypic and functional markers found at the surface or inside the cell or in the nucleus are used to assess the type of T cell response generated. (B) Discreet subsets of immunofluorescently stained cells are separated using fluorescence-activated cell sorting (FACS). Bulk or single cell transcriptomic work can be used to examine expression of all or targeted gene transcripts. At the single-cell level and using index sorting, integrative analysis combines protein expression data with transcriptomic analysis to provide extensive characterization of cellular heterogeneity.

of polyclonally stimulated CMV-specific, Flu-specific, and EBV-specific cells.[19] Despite such advances, our understanding of lymphocyte diversity is still limited, and the difficulty in retaining viable cells after mass cytometry hinders subsequent functional assays or transcriptomic analysis.

Another avenue to augment our understanding of immune responses at the cellular level is to deconvolute signals through more sophisticated computational analyses. For example, a combinatorial polyfunctionality analysis of antigen-specific T cell subsets (COMPASS), which calculates either a global or weighted polyfunctionality score, identified two antigen-specific CD4 + T cell subsets that were significantly correlated with infection risk and not identified in the initial, traditional correlates analysis of the RV144 HIV vaccine efficacy trial.[16]

In addition to the identification of cell subsets, flow cytometric methods can help catalog the vast array of secreted factors such as cytokines, chemokines and other proteins that condition the quality of the immune response induced by vaccination. These multiplexed microsphere suspension array-based immunoassays can simultaneously measure up to 500 analytes from serum, plasma, cerebrospinal fluid, mucosal samples and cell culture supernatant.[20] A better understanding of the signaling cascade that initiates the host response to vaccination would be a valuable tool toward developing vaccine strategies that better leverage the crosstalk between the innate and adaptive immune responses.

Metabolomics

Complementing the upstream transcriptomics, metabolomics offers a way to systematically analyze all small molecules or metabolites that are secreted in cells or tissues by host and microbial cells in response to an environmental stimulus. It combines mass spectrometry and nuclear magnetic resonance spectroscopy with biostatistics and mathematical modeling and has been applied to several metabolic diseases including diabetes and obesity.[21,22] It hold promise for vaccine research, as innate and adaptive immune responses are defined by changes in the set of metabolites within memory and effector cells. Additionally, metabolites from the gastrointestinal microbiome have been identified as important to cardiometabolic diseases.[23] Thus, one can envision that gut microbiota could emerge as an important factor for vaccine strategies against pathogens such as HIV-1 that disrupt mucosal immunity and the balance of intestinal flora. Because the metabolome reflects internal and environmental signals, metabolomics can help measure individual exposures as a way to discover the causes of diseases, thus bridging the persistent gap in our understanding of the mechanistic links between genotype and phenotype. When employed in large cohorts, metabolic profiling can be coupled with genome-wide association studies (GWAS) to elucidate the associations between single nucleotide polymorphisms and metabolites, or so-called metabolic quantitative trait loci (mQTL). Although there are typically multiple SNPs associated with a single metabolite and vice-versa, such studies could help characterize the etiology of protective immune responses in the context of vaccination.

Genomics

Given the important role of HLA alleles in the adaptive immune response, it is clear that genomic profiles would likely impact vaccine responsiveness. Several studies have examined mono- and dizygotic twins to identify the key genetic factors associated with vaccine responses. These studies demonstrated that the heritability of vaccine-induced antibody responses depending on the vaccine of study, ranging from 39% heritability for mumps to 89% for measles.[24–30] Interestingly, for some vaccines, the antibody responses were modulated or restricted by specific HLA alleles (class II for the TB bacilli calmette-guerin vaccine[26]; DRB1* locus for the hepatitis B virus (HBV) surface antigen recombinant subunit vaccine[25]; DPB1*13 for the HIV vectored/subunit (ALVAC/AIDSVAX) vaccine tested in the RV 144 trial[31]). The heterogeneity of genomic influence on different vaccines likely reflects the baseline genomic variation at a population level. This makes the characterization of vaccine responses, as a function of genomic profiling, a particularly complex enterprise. Most studies, even in large cohorts, can only detect very strong magnitudes of association. Small and thus underpowered studies are therefore inherently unreliable and often irreproducible. Meta-analyses can sometimes resolve these discrepancies, as in the case of HBV vaccination where an aggregate look at variants in class II HLA and interleukin-4 were found to significantly associate with robust antibody responses.[32]

Genomic analyses have also been used to identify genetic causes of vaccine failures: for example, individuals who are homozygous for the MAL/TIRAP Ser180Leu polymorphism have been found to carry a near sixfold higher risk of non-meningitic invasive *Haemophilus influenzae* type B (Hib) Hib disease following Hib vaccination.[33] A better understanding of B and T cell repertoires following vaccination, via high-throughput genetic sequencing, is another dividend of the growing interface between vaccinology and genomics. The fundamental challenge, however, is to translate these findings into the development of new vaccines that can be tailored to specific populations. Vaccines could also be adapted to the genetic determinants of the pathogen; as such, the analysis of breakthrough infections in vaccine efficacy trials, or sieve analysis can identify pathogen variants that are associated with increased or decreased vaccine efficacy.

Sieve Analysis

The principal way of deriving information from vaccine efficacy studies is through case-control analyses, whereby the immune responses elicited in vaccine recipients who became infected with the pathogen targeted by the vaccine are compared to vaccine recipients who did not become infected. An alternative method is called a "sieve analysis," which analyzes data only among those individuals who became infected, but compare them according to whether they received the vaccine or a placebo.[34] Sieve analyses have been most extensively performed for HIV vaccine efficacy trials.[35,36] The diversity of HIV sequences presents a significant challenge for HIV vaccine design and development, as each HIV infected individual possesses his or her own unique viral population. Although continued HIV diversification within populations and individuals poses a problem for the identification of optimal vaccine inserts, it also offers an opportunity to measure and understand the impact of a vaccine on HIV sequence diversity. Sieve analyses, however, can only be performed in placebo-controlled trials and if the trial was conducted properly (no interference, limited bias, participants remained blinded to their treatment assignment). This approach can identify responses that may correspond to the right target but failed to mediate protection because these responses were either not potent enough or suffered from immune interference. Sieve analyses can focus on specific genes, subgene loci, or subsequences from a sequencing read (i.e., k-mer) in order to dissect identify areas of immune pressure. The principal sieve effect that is identified could then be leveraged to block the establishment of infection in the vaccine group, by mechanisms that could restrict specific variants (i.e., those sequences that are the closest to the vaccine insert). Vaccine-induced immunity could also leave marks on pathogen genomes of pathogens, whereby sites that correspond to T cell or antibody epitopes show more mutations in the vaccine group than in the placebo group (Fig. 5.2). Innovative but pragmatic approaches will be needed to build on these findings to create effective vaccines.

Computational Analysis

All of the emerging high-throughput technologies must ultimately be integrated into an iterative cycle that links thousands of biological measurements to sophisticated computational analyses to be followed by experimental testing. Interpreting all these data still remains a complex task, not only because of the large number of parameters analyzed, but also because number of assay readouts are indirect surrogate measurements that represent multiple levels of immune response. The complexity of the accumulated "omics" data requires multivariate statistical methods that identify biological factors of relevance to various immunologic settings. A critical first step toward that end

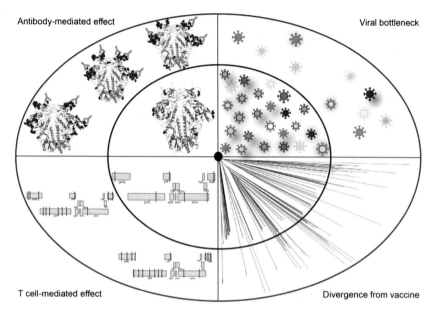

FIGURE 5.2   Schematic representation of sieve effects. The inner circle represents sequences from placebo recipients, the outer circle breakthrough sequences from vaccine recipients. Sieve effects are figured for HIV-1 (from the upper-right corner): the vaccine can block viruses from establishing infection (higher viral diversity in the placebo group); the vaccine can specifically block viruses that are more similar to the vaccine (extra-divergence from the vaccine in the vaccine group); the vaccine can mediate T cell responses that will drive mutations in T cell epitopes in the proteins that were included in the vaccine (here, Gag, Pol, and Nef); the vaccine can mediate humoral responses that will be associated with mutations at antibody footprints on the envelope protein.

involves the organization and curation of thousands of heterogeneous readouts that are likely to be biased by batch effects, variable degrees of noise and arbitrary decisions about what data to include (e.g., flow cytometric analysis depends on manual, subjective analyses of individual data files).

Coping with the high dimensionality of the data, whereby many variables are observed for a limited number of samples, is central to the analysis of systems data. While researchers must perform a priori power calculations to anticipate a sample size that will facilitate the detection of a signal in a multivariate setting, it has to be noted that in vaccine efficacy trials the limited number of samples will preclude certain types of analyses.

There is a caveat to be noted; that heterogeneous and multidimensional data sets can yield significant results by chance alone, requiring corrections for multiple testing (Bonferroni) or methods to control the false discovery rate (e.g., Benjamini & Hochberg). A standard practice for systems data is to summarize the information into a smaller data set. Different approaches exist to reduce data dimensionality; they rely on principal component analysis (PCA), clustering and machine learning methods, and a number of derivative methods (LDA, Canonical Correlation Analysis, Partial Least Squares regression). Conflicting outcomes have been described in the systems biology field, highlighting the need for further attention and research on standardization issues.[37]

It will be important to develop web-based tools to facilitate data mining and analysis of systems biology data. Some of these platforms should be dedicated to disseminate the full set of correlated measurements (beyond the salient results associated with a given publication). Transparency should increase the value of these systems vaccinology data sets and ensure enhanced discovery. Importantly, multilateral partnerships are needed between clinical investigators, researchers (in vitro and animal model experimentation), and computational biologists, and collaborative efforts are the most efficient way to generate and integrate comprehensive data sets to maximize knowledge and offer new opportunities to dissect mechanisms of vaccine-induced immunity.

CONCLUSION

The search for vaccines against pathogens such as HIV, malaria, and TB, has been hampered by the absence of robust correlates of protection and the ethical limitations on human challenge models (though progress is being made for malaria). Profiling the complex relationships between the different cell types and soluble factors is necessary to better understand the genesis, quality and kinetics of immune response that develop postvaccination. Systems vaccinology approaches promise to shed light on mechanistic insights that can be actionable for vaccine innovation. These large data sets generated with different "omics" platforms have helped define correlates of immunogenicity for several vaccines, a necessary precursor to the identification of correlates of protection. While the identification of universal features of vaccine protection is still a distant goal, there are still areas within systems vaccinology where tangible progress can be made in the next decade. For example, the field as a whole is moving closer to defining sets of factors that are associated with certain vaccine adverse events and discerning the specific contributions each component of a vaccine (e.g., platform, antigen, prime, boost, adjuvant) provides for the immune response. Additional areas of study, including glycomics and epigenetics, will also complement expanding applications of systems vaccinology. Recent studies are already demonstrating the breadth of influence that systems biology is having on vaccine research and development.[38,39] The expectation is that systematic approaches toward scientific investigation, using high-throughput (-OMICS) technologies coupled with sophisticated computation analysis of large data sets will recapitulate their successes in other areas of biomedicine and begin to reveal key to the molecular and cellular signatures of vaccine-induced immunity.

ACKNOWLEDGMENTS

We thank Drs. Shelly Krebs, Nelson Michael, and Lydie Trautmann for their critical review of this chapter.

DISCLAIMER

The views expressed are those of the authors and should not be construed to represent the positions of the US Army or the Department of Defense.

REFERENCES

1. Pulendran B, Li S, Nakaya HI. Systems vaccinology. *Immunity* 2010;**33**(4):516−29.
2. Li S, et al. Molecular signatures of antibody responses derived from a systems biology study of five human vaccines. *Nat Immunol* 2014;**15**(2):195−204.
3. Nakaya HI, et al. Systems biology of vaccination for seasonal influenza in humans. *Nat Immunol* 2011;**12**(8):786−95.
4. Chung AW, et al. Dissecting polyclonal vaccine-induced humoral immunity against HIV using systems serology. *Cell* 2015;**163**(4):988−98.
5. Zak DE, Tam VC, Aderem A. Systems-level analysis of innate immunity. *Annu Rev Immunol* 2014;**32**:547−77.
6. Querec TD, et al. Systems biology approach predicts immunogenicity of the yellow fever vaccine in humans. *Nat Immunol* 2009;**10**(1):116−25.
7. Bucasas KL, et al. Early patterns of gene expression correlate with the humoral immune response to influenza vaccination in humans. *J Infect Dis* 2011;**203**(7):921−9.
8. Haynes BF, et al. Immune-correlates analysis of an HIV-1 vaccine efficacy trial. *N Engl J Med* 2012;**366**(14):1275−86.
9. Sabchareon A, et al. Protective efficacy of the recombinant, live-attenuated, CYD tetravalent dengue vaccine in Thai schoolchildren: a randomised, controlled phase 2b trial. *Lancet* 2012;**380**(9853):1559−67.
10. Sirivichayakul C, et al. Plaque reduction neutralization antibody test does not accurately predict protection against dengue infection in Ratchaburi cohort, Thailand. *Virol J* 2014;**11**:48.
11. Villar L, et al. Efficacy of a tetravalent dengue vaccine in children in Latin America. *N Engl J Med* 2015;**372**(2):113−23.
12. Corey L, et al. Immune correlates of vaccine protection against HIV-1 acquisition. *Sci Transl Med* 2015;**7**(310):310rv7.
13. Robinson JP, Roederer M. HISTORY OF SCIENCE. Flow cytometry strikes gold. *Science* 2015;**350**(6262):739−40.
14. Baumgarth N, Roederer M. A practical approach to multicolor flow cytometry for immunophenotyping. *J Immunol Methods* 2000;**243**(1−2):77−97.
15. Perfetto SP, Chattopadhyay PK, Roederer M. Seventeen-colour flow cytometry: unravelling the immune system. *Nat Rev Immunol* 2004;**4**(8):648−55.
16. Lin L, et al. COMPASS identifies T-cell subsets correlated with clinical outcomes. *Nat Biotechnol* 2015;**33**(6):610−16.
17. Bendall SC, et al. Single-cell mass cytometry of differential immune and drug responses across a human hematopoietic continuum. *Science* 2011;**332**(6030):687−96.
18. Bendall SC, et al. A deep profiler's guide to cytometry. *Trends Immunol* 2012;**33**(7):323−32.

19. Newell EW, et al. Cytometry by time-of-flight shows combinatorial cytokine expression and virus-specific cell niches within a continuum of CD8 + T cell phenotypes. *Immunity* 2012;**36**(1):142–52.

20. Lin A, Salvador A, Carter JM. Multiplexed microsphere suspension array-based immunoassays. *Methods Mol Biol* 2015;**1318**:107–18.

21. Wang TJ, et al. Metabolite profiles and the risk of developing diabetes. *Nat Med* 2011;**17**(4):448–53.

22. Wurtz P, et al. Metabolic signatures of adiposity in young adults: Mendelian randomization analysis and effects of weight change. *PLoS Med* 2014;**11**(12):e1001765.

23. Neves AL, et al. The microbiome and its pharmacological targets: therapeutic avenues in cardiometabolic diseases. *Curr Opin Pharmacol* 2015;**25**:36–44.

24. Lee YC, et al. Influence of genetic and environmental factors on the immunogenicity of Hib vaccine in Gambian twins. *Vaccine* 2006;**24**(25):5335–40.

25. Hohler T, et al. Differential genetic determination of immune responsiveness to hepatitis B surface antigen and to hepatitis A virus: a vaccination study in twins. *Lancet* 2002;**360**(9338):991–5.

26. Newport MJ, et al. Genetic regulation of immune responses to vaccines in early life. *Genes Immun* 2004;**5**(2):122–9.

27. Tan PL, et al. Twin studies of immunogenicity – determining the genetic contribution to vaccine failure. *Vaccine* 2001;**19**(17–19):2434–9.

28. Klein NP, et al. A role for genetics in the immune response to the varicella vaccine. *Pediatr Infect Dis J* 2007;**26**(4):300–5.

29. Konradsen HB, et al. The influence of genetic factors on the immune response as judged by pneumococcal vaccination of mono- and dizygotic Caucasian twins. *Clin Exp Immunol* 1993;**92**(3):532–6.

30. Brodin P, et al. Variation in the human immune system is largely driven by non-heritable influences. *Cell* 2015;**160**(1–2):37–47.

31. Prentice HA, et al. HLA class II genes modulate vaccine-induced antibody responses to affect HIV-1 acquisition. *Sci Transl Med* 2015;**7**(296):296ra112.

32. Cui W, et al. Association of polymorphisms in the interleukin-4 gene with response to hepatitis B vaccine and susceptibility to hepatitis B virus infection: a meta-analysis. *Gene* 2013;**525**(1):35–40.

33. Ladhani SN, et al. Association between single-nucleotide polymorphisms in Mal/TIRAP and interleukin-10 genes and susceptibility to invasive haemophilus influenzae serotype b infection in immunized children. *Clin Infect Dis* 2010;**51**(7):761–7.

34. Edlefsen PT, Gilbert PB, Rolland M. Sieve analysis in HIV-1 vaccine efficacy trials. *Curr Opin HIV AIDS* 2013;**8**(5):432–6.

35. Rolland M, et al. Genetic impact of vaccination on breakthrough HIV-1 sequences from the STEP trial. *Nat Med* 2011;**17**(3):366–71.

36. Rolland M, et al. Increased HIV-1 vaccine efficacy against viruses with genetic signatures in Env V2. *Nature* 2012;**490**(7420):417–20.

37. Liquet B, et al. A novel approach for biomarker selection and the integration of repeated measures experiments from two assays. *BMC Bioinformatics* 2012;**13**:325.

38. Nakaya HI, et al. Systems analysis of immunity to influenza vaccination across multiple years and in diverse populations reveals shared molecular signatures. *Immunity* 2015;**43**(6):1186–98.

39. Bartel J, et al. The human blood metabolome-transcriptome interface. *PLoS Genet* 2015;**11**(6):e1005274.

Chapter 6

Immunogenetics and Vaccination

M. John[1,2], S. Gaudieri[1,2,3] and S. Mallal[1,3]

[1]Murdoch University, Murdoch, WA, Australia, [2]University of Western Australia, Crawley, WA, Australia, [3]Vanderbilt University, Nashville, TN, United States

Humans and their primate ancestors have triumphed over many infectious diseases by virtue of immunological mechanisms which kill pathogens or co-adapt with commensals. A large part of this evolutionary success is the maintenance of genetic polymorphism in populations. It is notable therefore that genetic variation is almost universally discussed as a problem in the vaccine discourse. Organisms that utilize highly conserved and canonical proteins in the immune interactome are more likely to hijack host cellular processes, replicate, persist, and transmit to more individual hosts within a population. Inter-individual polymorphism, particularly in those proteins which present diverse microbial antigens to the immune system, has been critical for protecting individuals from such organisms and as a result have underpinned natural and vaccine-induced herd immunity for many past and present infectious diseases. However, as these forces operate at the level of specific host—pathogen interactions, it is not unexpected that poor response or adverse effects to otherwise successful vaccines for some individuals in a population is genetically determined and therefore predictable to some extent. Though there are examples of design iterations in licensed vaccines to provide dose, valency, or immunogen variations to specific subgroups and broaden population coverage, to date such adjustments have not been based on specified genetic variation. Investigational vaccines that remain the most challenging are against those pathogens which have successful adaptations to human immunity, including its polymorphisms. A central concept for immunogenetics is that for all pathogens, variation in the human leukocyte antigen (HLA) loci restricts not only the vaccine epitopes which are intracellularly processed and presented but also the breadth of the mature T cell repertoires that can be induced within

Human Vaccines: Emerging Technologies in Design and Development.
DOI: http://dx.doi.org/10.1016/B978-0-12-802302-0.00005-4

any individual because of the role of HLA in early life thymic education. These include the repertoires of CD4 T cells which influence effector, memory and regulatory T cell functions and B cell function, and CD8 T cells. HLA-peptide complexes also engage NK cells and dendritic cells through direct ligation of specific receptors, which also display polymorphism. Furthermore, in pathogens capable of antigenic drift, HLA or other polymorphic loci impacts the degree of similarity between the vaccine immunogen and circulating transmissible viruses imprinted by immune evasion from previous hosts. These multiplicative impacts mean that vaccine immunogenetics occupies a much wider landscape than single gene polymorphisms which influence vaccine antibody levels or antigen-specific IFNγ release in vaccine nonresponders. Some of the most difficult problems in new vaccine design such as population and individual-level immunodominance and pathogen diversity are strongly linked to human immunogenetic variation. Overcoming these issues by personalization requires an appreciation of why this variation has been optimized by human evolution, and then driven distinct evolutionary solutions in human pathogens.

IMMUNOGENETIC VARIATION

In-bred monomorphic animal models have contributed enormously to the understanding of fundamental immunology and the discipline of vaccinology. Translating knowledge of biological phenomena gained from such models to the clinical phase of vaccine development is frequently related to a central difference between such mice and men: humans are diverse. The vast expansion of genetic information derived from the International HapMap project, the 1000 genomes project and genome wide association (GWAS) studies over the last decade has shown the remarkable polyallelism of genes encoding proteins of the human immune system, between and even within populations with shared ancestries.[1-3] Associations between human gene variants and host susceptibility to acquisition or disease progression of infectious diseases have led to discoveries of important biological mechanisms in antimicrobial defense.

The Major Histocompatibility Complex

More than twenty years before the GWAS explosion, the prominence of immunogenetic polymorphism was evident in studies of the major histocompatibility complex (MHC), in which the cluster of HLA and non-HLA genes involved in myriad immunological pathways were shown to conform to conserved, "frozen" haplotypic structures and inherited en bloc but containing sites of intense polymorphism within, and between, genes.[4] The striking microanatomy of so many immunity-associated genes squeezed into a segment representing 0.1% of the human genome suggested common ancestral sequences and a dynamic evolutionary history marked by rapid diversification mechanisms such as cycles of local within-MHC segmental duplication events, inter-allele recombinations and indels, including insertions related to human endogenous retroviruses.[5] These studies were prescient in many ways, as much of the same phenomena have been found to apply to other eukaryotic multigene families, however the polymorphism of MHC remains comparatively extreme. It was Doherty and Zinkernagel, soon after their seminal discovery of HLA as antigen presenting molecules in the 1970s, who first proposed an adaptive basis for HLA polymorphism, based on the enhanced T cell surveillance associated with heterozygosity in the homologous murine H-2 system.[6] Since that time, a vast literature has debated the relative contributions of overdominant selection (heterozygote advantage), negative frequency dependant selection[7−9] and more recently, "associative balancing complex" evolution[10] for maintaining the allelic architecture of MHC. In a general sense, the evidence that the MHC has been subject to Darwinian selection pressures throughout millennia of vertebrate and human evolution derives from a number of consistent observations: there is an excess of HLA alleles maintained at intermediate frequencies in human populations, many alleles have been maintained over deep time (including some from early introgressions of DNA from Neandertals and Denisovans to modern humans and others pre-dating hominoid speciation), allele distribution differs between populations with different ancestral geographic origins and microbial environments (also a function of early migration histories and founder effects), blocks of linked alleles with putative epistasis in immune responses appear conserved despite adjacent recombination, and finally, non-synonymous nucleotide substitutions are preferentially distributed in exons coding peptide-binding regions of HLA molecules.[11,12] The peptide binding regions determine the microbial epitope repertoire, however other regions may be subject to selection based on indirect effects on the repertoire such as sites which regulate HLA surface expression.[13] In a genome which averages one to three high frequency alleles per gene (with the remainder being uncommon to rare variants), the current global allele counts for classical class I genes HLA-A is 3107, HLA-B 3887, and HLA class II HLA-DRB1 1829 (http://www.ebi.ac.uk/imgt/hla).

Genetic Variation in Non-MHC Loci

Microbial selection may be the basis for the lesser variation in other loci relevant to human immunity, such as the killer cell immunoglobulin-like receptor (KIR) family which displays dominant haplogroups, the closely linked leukocyte immunoglobulin-like receptors (LIRs), chemokines such as IL-10, and chemokine receptors such as CCR5. Despite evidence of selection, there have been very few cases of proven selection by particular pathogens, perhaps reflecting the distant time in which such influences operated and the incomplete knowledge of past epidemics and their social contexts in terms of human migrations and all competing selection forces. Selection and maintenance of a 32 base pair deletion in CCR5 in European-ancestry populations by past epidemics such as the bubonic plague and smallpox have been explored and debated but not ultimately proven,[14] while data on the deleterious effect of the mutation on the clinical severity of West Nile virus encephalitis suggests the possibility of highly pathogen-specific effects in past evolution.[15,16] Coevolution of specific KIR-HLA-C ligand receptor pairs in diverse populations has been associated with selective effects of Malaria.[17]

IMMUNOGENETIC ASSOCIATIONS WITH INFECTIONS AND VACCINES

Population diversity means, *eo ipso*, that there will be individuals within a population that carry alleles which are less successful or functional for any one particular pathogen. This is the general basis of the relatively small number of reported unfavorable genetic associations with infectious diseases, such as HLA-B*35 subtypes and faster HIV associated CD4 T cell decline,[18] HLA-A*24 and influenza A-associated mortality,[19] various HLA class I alleles and SARS susceptibility,[20,21] multiple HLA and non-HLA alleles, and Dengue disease severity[22] to name a few. Interestingly, alleles that are more successful or protective against a pathogen now may owe their success to ancestral primate alleles which had been subject to positive selection by a related pathogen, in a case of history repeating itself. It is notable that the more favorable control of HIV viremia is associated with carriage of HLA-B*57:01, -B*57:03, -B*58:01, and -B*27:05[23] which happen to be the alleles which share the most transpecies polymorphisms in exon 2−3 peptide-binding coding regions with the relatively restricted array of chimpanzee (patr) MHC class I genotypes compared with all other population HLA-B alleles.[24] These are also most likely to bind more evolutionary conserved epitopes in HIV-1.[24,25] These data support analyses demonstrating the similarity between SIV epitope repertoires of Patr MHC and those individuals with nonprogressive HIV-1 infection.[26] This suggests that it is preferential binding of evolutionary conserved epitopes similar to those of extant MHC alleles after the selective sweep in chimpanzees[27] which underpins more suppressive CD8 T cells responses against HIV.

As vaccines are designed to recapitulate infection in a nonpathogenic way, a genetic influence on vaccine responses and protection from pathogen challenge is not unexpected. Studies have reported genetic associations of various known correlates of protection or readouts of immunogenicity induced by licensed vaccines against Hepatitis A and B, measles, mumps, rubella, influenza, smallpox, *Streptococcus pneumoniae*, *Neisseria meningitides*, *Haemophilus influenza*, diphtheria, tetanus, and tuberculosis, though there is a marked inequality in the number of studies examining these different vaccines and pathogens.[28,29] Relative to the vast literature on other disease associations, vaccine-gene associations remain relatively understudied as they have relied heavily on postlicensure sampling, and not as part of vaccine development in clinical trial populations. The reported vaccine response associations to date have not had an equal chance of being verified in independent studies, as particular vaccines have been the subject of genetic association studies more frequently than others. Vaccines against pathogens which are high public health threats, priorities for eradication, highly transmissible or displaying significant heterogeneity in population responses should attract greater scientific interest and investment in genetic association research. However operational considerations such as the ability to easily ascertain a defined cohort of vaccinees in the community such as in occupational or educational settings and availability of standardized correlates of protection (such as antibody titers) by routine assays may be significant drivers of feasibility. There is a relative abundance of studies on the response to recombinant hepatitis B surface antigen vaccine, measles, and rubella for example. Table 6.1 collates genetic associations with vaccine responses which have been replicated in two or more independent populations, acknowledging that this is fundamentally skewed by the extent to which studies have examined the same set of genetic loci using the same methods, for the same outcome measures, in genetically comparable and powered vaccinee populations. The stringency of p-value criteria for significance is also not comparable between studies of different sizes and with different approaches to multiple test correction.

Notwithstanding the heterogeneity in study designs and populations, a few consistent associations involving HLA genotypes, cytokines and complement proteins have been reported.[29-49] Some associations are more robust than others in terms of strength of association (odds ratio), significance value and reproducibility. Aside from the study design issues mentioned above, analytical techniques have evolved from early twin studies, limited candidate gene type or single nucleotide polymorphism (SNP) association studies, extended SNP arrays to more recent GWAS, accompanied by advances in analytical methods to adjust associations for multiple comparisons and linkage disequilibrium, the latter being a prominent issue for any HLA or non-HLA associations in the MHC. These developments have made apparent the extent to which differential immunogenicity of many vaccines, as with natural infection, is highly multigenic with many loci contributing significant but small incremental effects at the population level. Notably, accumulated data from twin studies and studies of HLA genotype associations and candidate immune gene SNPs was estimated to explain only 30% of inter-individual variability in measles antibody responses.[40] As vaccine development moves from the relative empiricism of Pasteur's rules of "isolate, inactivate, and inject" to an iterative enterprise, guided by high dimensional genomics and other "omics" analysis,

TABLE 6.1 Selected Consistent Genetic Associations With Outcomes of Current Vaccines

Vaccine	Genetic Association	Vaccine Outcome	Analysis Methods	Reference
HBV vaccine	HLA-DR3, -DR3 haplotypes, DRB1*03	Reduced/nonresponse	Candidate gene, family, and twin studies	30–32, 35
	HLA-DRB1*07	Reduced/nonresponse	Candidate gene, family, and twin studies	30–32
	C4Q0 alleles and haplotypes	Reduced or nonresponse	Candidate gene, family, and twin studies	33,34
	IL-12B	Reduced or nonresponse	Candidate gene, family, and twin studies	
	HLA-DR locus SNPs	Antibody nonresponse	Large scale SNP analysis > 6000 snps, 900 immune response genes	36
	CD11a/ITGAL	Peak antibody levels	Large scale SNP analysis in non-MHC genes large Gambian population	37
	HLA-DP1*05:01 and other HLA-DP loci SNPs	Response to booster vaccine	Case-control study	38
	HLA-DP loci SNP	Long term memory to infant vaccination	GWAS	38
Measles	HLA-DQA1*02:01	Antibody response	Candidate gene (HLA) studies using two independant cohorts	39

	HLA-B08:01	Measles-specific IFNγ	Candidate gene (HLA) studies using two independant cohorts	40
	CD46 (measles receptor)	Antibody response	Candidate gene studies	41–43
	SLAM	Antibody response	Candidate gene studies	41,42
	IL2	Cellular responses (IFNγ)	Candidate gene/SNP studies	44,45
	IL10	Cell responses	Candidate gene/SNP studies	44,45
	IL12RB1	Measles antibody and cellular responses	Candidate gene/SNP studies	46
Rubella	HLA-B*27:05, -DPB1*04:01	Rubella antibody	HLA genotyping and association study	47
	HLA-DPB1*04:01	Rubella antibody	GWAS	48
Smallpox	HLA-DQB1*03:02, -DRB1*04:03, -DRB1*08:01, -DRB1*15:01	Antibody and IFNγ responses	Candidate gene (HLA) studies	49

more genetic associations with well phenotyped immunological measurements and specific trial endpoints are likely to be discovered and verified for licensed and investigational vaccines. The value of genetic studies being part of phase 2/3 clinical trials is that rates of infection in vaccinees, as evidence of true vaccine failure, rather than various cocorrelates or biomarkers of protection, can be examined with much greater veracity than in postlicensing observational studies. An example is a study of the association between HLA-A*02 and vaccine efficacy in the RV144 HIV vaccine trial.[50]

It should be noted that the extent to which true associations would practically impact herd immunity or pathogen clearance at the population level depends also on the transmissibility of the pathogen. For example, the highly infectious measles virus may still cause outbreaks in vaccinated populations despite >94% vaccine efficacy[51] in the face of high load or super-spreader exposures, as recently reported.[52] On the otherhand, for less contagious pathogens, genetic determinants of low frequency or small effect size may not significantly impede the ability of vaccine to prevent disease in high prevalence epidemics.

FUNCTIONAL BASIS OF IMMUNOGENETIC ASSOCIATIONS WITH VACCINE RESPONSE

Some associations may have a relatively simple mechanistic and testable link to vaccine function. For example, CD46 is a complement regulatory protein but used by measles, HHV6 and Neisseria for cell entry. Polymorphism is relatively limited, however consistent associations between a CD46 intronic SNP and reduced serological and cellular responses to measles vaccination may reflect differential activation of interferon-gamma dependent pathways through this receptor.[53] The action of IL-12 is likely to be important in induction of these pathways and indeed a variant in the IL-12B gene which affects IL12 production is also associated with measles-specific responses.[46] Similarly, of the many immune evasion mechanisms adopted by pox-viruses, secretion of an IL-18 binding protein points to the importance of IL-18 and IL18R to antipoxvirus immunity and may explain observations that SNPs in the genes encoding these cytokines are associated with differential cellular responses to vaccinia-based small pox vaccination.[54] These types of specific interactions can point to key checkpoints within immune responses which can then be used to engineer relevant molecules into vaccines for delivery alongside the immunogen as novel adjuvants. Such interventions may increase the immunogenicity for the broader population, rather than just those rare individuals with the specific associated genotype.

In general, genes relevant to many cellular processes from cell entry to cytokine receptors have specialized functions in the immune response as a whole. They tend to be relatively ancestrally conserved and largely bi- or tri-allelic for major alleles, with perhaps a number of variants which are rare because of purifying selection. They are therefore most likely to have defined but small effects on global immunogenicity, most commonly by modifying the strength of certain activation signals within a large network of events. Associations with determinants in multigene families are more complicated and HLA in particular may exert effects on immunogenicity in a number of different ways.

HLA, Antigen Processing, and Epitope-Binding

The most obvious influence of HLA on vaccine immunogenicity is in the restriction of vaccine epitopes that are processed, stably transported and presented to antigen-specific T cells. The importance of the strength of stable HLA-peptide binding is evident in the well documented association between a group of specific HLA-B alleles and natural HIV control. A number of observational cohort studies had implicated HLA-B*27:05, HLA-B*57:01, and the similar alleles HLA-B*57:03 and −HLA-B*58:01 most consistently. These have been subsequently confirmed in several GWAS including one which showed that HIV control was mediated by specific amino acid positions within the peptide binding groove of HLA-B.[23] Position 97 forming the C pocket of the HLA-B peptide binding cleft was most strongly associated with antiviral control in this study, highlighting the importance of the HLA-peptide interaction to the efficacy of the immune response. Separate lines of evidence based on the preference for arginine at the P1 and P2 anchor positions of HLA-B27-restricted epitopes and tryptophan at the c-terminus of HLA-B57 restricted epitopes suggest that these HLAs are unique in binding such epitopes so stably, which may contribute to strong immunodominance of these epitope-specific responses within individuals. These preferences are also likely to structurally constrain the epitopes from mutation and cause costs to replicative capacity once mutated under immune pressure.[55−57] This natural mechanism appears to be equally relevant to the T cell responses elicited by the MRKAd5 HIV-1 gag/pol/nef vaccine tested in the STEP trial, as determined by a GWAS of IFNγ Elispot responses measured in trial participants.[58] As previously discussed, the benefits of these binding preferences parallel those of analogous MHC alleles in the natural primate hosts of SIV,[24−26] as well as being observed in the experimental SIV macaque model.[55]

Not all HLA associations may be mediated by characteristics of their peptide binding regions only. Four independent HIV GWASs provided the first evidence for a novel role for level of surface expression of HLA-C in HIV control.[23,59−61] This led to functional studies showing that HLA-C expression is subject to strong post-transcriptional regulation by microRNAs which bind to the polymorphic 3'UTR of the HLA-C gene.[62,63] This interaction regulates levels of endogenous HLA-C levels at the cell surface and

HLA-C expression levels predict HIV outcomes independently of protective HLA-B alleles in both European and African-American cohorts. Finally, high expressing HLA-C allotypes induce more escape mutations evident in HIV sequences[13,64] suggesting stronger HLA-C restricted CD8 T cell selective pressure.

HLA and the T Cell Repertoire

Beyond mechanisms associated with immunogen-derived peptide processing and presentation, HLA fundamentally predetermines the CD4 and CD8 T cell receptor (TCR) repertoire and the spectrum of T cell affinities within an antigen-specific response available to respond to any vaccine. This follows from self-protein determinants being presented in the context of HLA in thymic epithelium in early life. The education of immature T cells is contingent upon proliferation of specific T cell clones which have a sufficient level of binding to HLA-self peptide complexes, and activation induced apoptosis of those which are too strongly self-reactive. Thus, through a process involving both positive clonal selection and negative clonal deletion, HLA shapes the mature TCR view of the "immunological self" as well as pathogenic nonself in a way that is unique to each individual. At the population level, analysis of peptide similarities between HIV and human proteins has shown a rate of similarity, in significant part driven by HIV-HERV similarity, and an inverse correlation between immunogenicity of HIV peptides in population Elispot screening and similarity of those peptides to host-derived peptides, as expected for a mature T cell immunome trained to discriminate self from nonself at the peptide level.[65] Could HLA have allele-specific effects on the TCR repertoire which differentially impacts infection (or vaccine) outcome? Once again in the HIV field, it has been proposed that HLA-B57 and -B27 bind a smaller array of self peptides compared with other HLAs and are therefore less subject to thymic negative clonal deletion, making them more cross-reactive to HIV escape variants and perhaps more prone to autoimmunity.[66]

Biases in TCR recruitment may further determine immunogenicity within a given HLA-restriction. Studies of TCR usage associated with anti-HIV responses restricted by a single HLA genotype suggest the dominant engagement of particular public TCRs determines immunodominant responses[67] and studies of an immunodominant HLA-B27-restricted HIV response has shown that TCRs which were more cross reactive to escape variants distinguished those with viral control from noncontrollers.[68]

T Cell Immunodominance

These data are all naturally relevant to the issue of immunodominance, which characterizes both CD4 and CD8 T cell responses and can be a difficult problem in vaccine design, especially for pathogens whose natural hierarchies of immunodominance are clearly not effective in most cases. Originally applied to the antigen-specific CD4 T cell responses of in-bred model systems in the context of a few viruses, it was recognized that the majority of antigen-specific T cells detected in a primary immune response within an individual are directed against a dominant fraction of all possible epitopes potentially derived from the viral proteome. Immunodominance at the individual level is a consistent feature of the human immune response against a wide array of small and complex pathogens, as demonstrated for influenza, HIV, CMV, hepatitis B and C, among others. A number of factors have been shown to impact immunodominance at the individual level. In the case of CD8+ antiviral T cell responses, the kinetics of viral protein expression (late vs early expressed proteins) in infected cells, size, stability and cellular localization of different proteins, pathogen evasion mechanisms to block processing in infected cells and inhibit direct priming (as perfected by CMV), the route of infection or vaccination and the original primary or heterologous memory responses from past pathogen exposures may all influence which epitope-specific T cells dominate the global antiviral T cell response. It has been reported that more than 90% of immunodominance in antiviral responses can be explained by only 1% of potential peptides having sufficient binding affinity to the expressed HLA class I molecules and able to reach the required threshold level of total antigen presentation to activate a primary CD8 T cell response.[69] Recently a cell-free HLA class II antigen processing system has suggested that HLA-DR, HLA-DM along with endo and exo-peptidases alone can largely account for selection of peptides from complex antigens, including vaccine immunogens.[70]

Because of these effects on antigen processing, presentation and activation as well as on naive and memory T cell repertoires at the individual level, HLA imposes a significant restriction to the number of epitopes ultimately targeted, relative to the number of potential epitopes available to target. Yet, HLA underpins both tolerance to self and immunity to many diverse pathogens, suggesting that the choice of epitopes is highly strategic. This begs the question, what properties of potential epitope sequences confer a strategic advantage to HLA alleles, and drive HLA evolution? In 1995, Hughes and Hughes hypothesized that MHC adaptively binds evolutionarily conserved hydrophobic peptides, resulting in effective self-non-self discrimination and reduced likelihood of pathogen escape over a broad range of pathogens.[71] A large scale bioinformatic analyses of binding affinities of HLA-A and -B alleles and evolutionary conservation of human and viral proteomes across 52 viral families supported this generalized view, and further showed that variations in the degree of binding to evolutionary conserved elements (termed targeting efficiency) was HLA locus, allele and virus-dependant, in keeping with specific host-viral coadaptive relationships.[24] That is, though targeting evolutionary conserved elements of viral proteins is a general property of HLA class I, there is a distribution of varying targeting efficiencies across individual HLA alleles within each locus for any one particular virus. Hence, HLA-A and few selected HLA-B alleles, such as HLA-B57 and -B58, displayed the greatest average efficiencies for DNA viruses with longer histories of human coadaption such as herpesviruses and adenoviruses. In evolutionary terms, the "newer" HLA-B locus alleles displayed higher average targeting efficiencies against RNA viruses. While identifying global trends, the application to individual viral-host relationships have been remarkably predictive, including the broad link between HLA-B and HIV immune selection, and the association of HLA-B*57 group alleles in particular to conserved epitope targets in HIV-1 *Gag* and viral control, as discussed above. Individual-specific efficiency scores (based on HLA-A and -B genotype) also predicted influenza A H1NI-specific T cell responses and mortality.[19] A notable case to investigate are flaviviruses, for which HLA class I generally appeared to favor targeting nonconserved elements. In this context, the targeting efficiency of specific HLA alleles and dengue virus proteins predicted risk of dengue hemorrhagic fever and this was postulated to be a function of T cell responses against nonconserved elements being more cross-reactive in secondary infection.[24] This and many other intriguing virus-specific patterns of HLA class I-restriction raised in these analyses have not been fully explored, but should be. It is only through the lens of evolution, that the deterministic nature of immunodominance in natural infection can be understood and predicted for new vaccine design. Furthermore, this explains why the MHC and associated proteins appears pivotal to immune evasion for so many viruses, and mechanisms will vary depending on viral intrinsic constraints. For all human herpesviruses, this includes the approach of limiting protein expression by latency or encoding proteins with "host shut-off" functions virtually along the entire HLA-class I peptide presentation pathway.[72] In striking contrast, HIV-1 may actively exploit the property of immunodominance by its induction of early cytotoxic immunodominant responses which rapidly select escape mutations and shift T cell responses to other subdominant and variable epitopes, gradually inflating particular T cell specificities in chronic infection but without effective viral inhibition.[73–75]

HLA and Induction of Natural Killer Cells and Dendritic Cells

It is worth remembering that HLA may mediate differential immune responses through effector mechanism others than T cells, including those potentially inducible by vaccines against viruses. The polymorphic KIRs modulate NK cell activity through detection of missing HLA class I, as a signal of intracellular viral infection or cancer transformation and a number of specific interactive associations between KIR-HLA with HIV disease outcomes[76] and KIR alleles and HIV sequence variation have been characterized.[77] HLA interaction with some of the 11 LILRs expressed on lymphoid and myeloid lineage cells is another potentially relevant interaction and has been explored in explaining HIV disease progression associated with HLA-B*35:02 and −B*35:03.[78]

HLA, KIR, and Pathogen Diversity

Successful vaccines prior to the 1970s did not have to engage significantly with issues of antigenic variation to a great extent (e.g., against invariant small pox, yellow fever, measles, mumps, rubella associated pathogens). The standard approaches to diversity since then has been to either match the composition of immunogens with dominant strains, increasing the valency of serotype-specific capsular antigens, e.g., in vaccines against *S. pneumoniae*, *N. meningitides*, or periodically reformulating vaccine antigens in response to new antigenic clusters, such as for Influenza A virus vaccine. In each case, the dominant mechanism(s) of antigenic diversity generation depends on intrinsic pathogen-specific characteristics and selection imposed by immune and nonimmune host factors.[79] For the most part, diversity considerations for most bacteria, protozoans such as *Plasmodium falciperum* and many common viruses center on the interaction between surface or capsular antigens or glycoproteins with antibodies, in which the genetic influence on antigen binding specificity is primarily through somatic cell recombination and hypermutation, rather than in the germ line cell, although HLA class II would restrict the cognate CD4 T cell responses that provide help to B cells.

The diversity problem in relation to small RNA viruses such as HIV and HCV is orders of magnitude more extreme, owing to the presence of error-prone polymerases, rapid replication cycles and, in the case of HIV, high intracellular recombination rate. HCV has a much higher replication rate than HIV, an additional error rate from requiring positive to negative, and negative to positive strand transcription and the absence of any constraint imposed by overlapping open reading frames. These characteristics provide the evolutionary basis for selection and fixation of mutations which escape antigen-specific antiviral responses mediated by HLA-restricted T cells and KIR-restricted NK cells. Since the phenomenon of HIV escape from CD8 T cell responses was first described,[80] an extensive literature has documented its occurrence longitudinally in acute and early infection, chronic infection, in both structural and accessory HIV proteins, at sites subject to antiretroviral drug selection and in response to vaccine-induced responses in animals and humans.[81] It was the studies that examined escape at the population level however, that fully revealed the remarkable plasticity of HIV as a pathogen of human populations, showing the extent to which circulating strains vary in a HLA allele-specific manner and therefore that HIV can retain or even increase in-vivo fitness in the context of a great diversity of HLA-restricted responses.[82] These types of studies have since shown that HLA drives whole mutational networks in HIV genomes, comprising primary and secondary/compensatory mutations and these are conditioned by subtype context.[83]

Even subtle differences between closely related HLA subtypes with identical peptide binding motifs influence escape pathways differently,[84,85] such that HIV diversity has characteristic profiles specific for particular ethnic/ancestry groups as a result of the prominent influence of HLA.[85] Analyses of single founder outbreaks have confirmed the significant contribution of HLA, especially the HLA-B locus to subsequent diversification of HIV.[86] Population-based approaches were used to identify the first evidence of KIR associated selection of HIV sequence variation.[77] Although there may be transmission-associated genetic bottlenecks which contract the range of potential transmitting strains, these data indicate that the ability of a single vaccine immunogen to prevent infection and/or avoid rapid viral escape after infection may be significantly impacted by host immunogenetics through effects on pathogen diversity.

IMMUNOGENETICS, VACCINE DESIGN, AND PERSONALIZATION

The recognition of genetically determined effects on vaccine immunogenicity have naturally led to consideration of personalized vaccinology, acknowledging key achievements in pharmacogenomics in recent years.[87] Given the varied ways in which vaccine efficacy or adverse effects may be predicted by host genotypes, what is the likelihood that vaccine design or delivery could be truly personalized? Though there are examples of vaccines (e.g., influenza, malaria) which have formulations which provide dose, valency or immunogen variations to specific subgroups and broaden population coverage, to date such adjustments have not been based explicitly on individual host, or even population-specific genetic variation. Better predictions could certainly be attractive for those publicized, serious adverse reactions which may be rare but in which the perceived risk in the community is problematic and leads to reduced vaccine uptake.

To understand the particular alignment of factors required to successfully translate immunogenetics to personalized medicine, the example of HLA-B*57:01 based use of the antiretroviral agent abacavir for treatment of HIV infection is instructive. Carriage of this allele has a positive predictive value for a potentially life threatening hypersensitivity reaction of 55%. However it is the 100% negative predictive value proven definitely in prospective controlled, randomized studies, some years after the strong association itself was first described,[88] which led to incorporation into the clinical practice guidelines of regulatory authorities and prescriber groups and widespread adoption of the test.[89,90] Availability of high quality laboratory services with adequate quality assurance and reimbursement as well as studies of cost-effectiveness further cemented HLA-B*57:01 testing as standard of care. Similar negative predictive values apply to screening of HLA-B*15:02 to prevent carbamazepine associated Stevens-Johnson syndrome/toxic epidermal necrolysis and

HLA-B*58:01 allopurinol adverse severe skin reactions but only in certain high risk groups such as those with Asian ancestry. However, the lower positive predictive values in both cases do lead to greater numbers of patients being denied these drugs unnecessarily. Other associations between drug adverse reactions and genetic loci may be strong and robust, but the predictive values are such that the numbers required to screen to avoid a single reaction are too high to be worthwhile in terms of cost and logistics as routine practice. The feasibility of genetic testing for specific markers relevant to vaccine administration is therefore a complex equation, and does not necessarily follow from the presence of strong genetic associations *per se*. To date, no single genetic associations with vaccine response or serious adverse reactions approach the predictive values or cost-effectiveness required for prevaccination screening. This may change with systems biology approaches which can identify a network of determinants that are sufficiently predictive of response or adverse reactions to guide vaccination feasibly.[91]

For new vaccine discovery and development, immunogenetic associations involving vaccine responses or natural infection can reveal biological mechanisms which can be incorporated into the design of adjuvants or specific formulations to increase immunogenicity. A greater investment in genetic studies earlier in vaccine development, rather than in postlicensing phases, would potentially guide development earlier making vaccines safer and more effective by the time of eventual licensure. The fact that antigenic diversity in certain pathogens is not just stochastic in nature but partly adaptive to avoid HLA or KIR-restricted cellular immunity is the rationale for development of vaccine immunogens explicitly designed to include conserved sequences. This aligns well with the evolutionary importance of conservation in general as a driver of HLA evolution and specialization of loci and specific allele-disease relationships. While the principle that vaccine induced immune responses against conserved areas within founder viruses would avoid infection by "preadapted" strains and suppress early escape after infection is almost self-evident, it is the precise design criteria for conservation or constraint that may determine the success of such approaches practically. In particular, there are few long subsegments in HIV population sequences, even within structurally important proteins such as Gag, which are absolutely conserved or exempt from selection pressure of *any* HLA allele. Indeed HIV adaptation to pandemic human infection would predict this to be the case. Nevertheless, candidate conserved HIV vaccines have been shown to be immunogenic, and recently use of anatomically isolated polyvalent vaccinations has shown promise in potentially focusing immune responses to conserved regions.[92] Finally novel vaccines could counteract problematic host polymorphism in the adaptive immune response by using vectors or adjuvants which can engage less polymorphic factors within the innate immune system or nonclassical antigen-presenting molecules which are largely monomorphic. While this strategy is attractive for adaptable pathogens in one sense, it also runs the risk of imposing a strong selecting pressure for strains that escape host monomorphism and abrogate vaccine efficacy across the whole population. This once again underscores the fact that host genetic polymorphism is protective for microbial defense at the population level, if at the expense of particular individuals. Rather than thought of just as a problem to overcome, immunogenetics is probably most important as a probe of biological mechanisms in pathogen-specific immunity which reflect human and pathogen coevolution. The aim of vaccines should be to recapitulate or harness evolutionarily successful strategies evident in natural models of protective immunity where these are present, and avoid or block the evolutionary solutions of pathogens in causing human disease. Genetic studies should continue to be an integral part of vaccine discovery and development, informed by an appreciation of the central place of the MHC and other highly polymorphic loci in many aspects of individualized vaccine responses.

REFERENCES

1. The International HapMap 3 Consortium. Integrating common and rare genetic variation in diverse human populations. *Nature* 2010;**467**:52−8.
2. Abecasis GR, et al. An integrated map of genetic variation from 1,092 human genomes. *Nature* 2012;**491**:56−65.
3. Hindorff LA, MacArthur J, Morales J, Junkins HA, Hall PN, Klemm AK, et al. *A catalog of published genome-wide association studies*. Available at: www.genome.gov/gwastudies.
4. Dawkins RL, Degli-Esposti MP, Abraham LJ, Zhang W, Christiansen FT. *Conservation versus polymorphism of the MHC in relation to transplantation, immune responses and autoimmune disease. Molecular evolution of the major histocompatibility complex*, vol. 59. NATO ASI Series; 1991. p. 391−402.
5. Dawkins R, Leelayuwat C, Gaudieri S, Tay G, Hui J, Gattley S, et al. Genomics of the major histocompatibility complex: haplotypes, duplication, retroviruses and disease. *Immunol Rev* 1999;**Vol. 167**:275−304.
6. Doherty PC, Zinkernagel R. Enhanced immune surveillance in mice heterozygous at the H-2 gene complex. *Nature* 1975;**256**:50−2.
7. Yeager M, Hughes AL. Evolution of the mammalian MHC: natural selection, recombination, and convergent evolution. *Immunol Rev* 1999;**167**:45−58.
8. Carrington M, Nelson GW, Martin MP, Kissner T, Vlahov D, Goedert JJ, et al. HLA and HIV-1: heterozygote advantage and B*35-Cw*04 disadvantage. *Science* 1999;**283**:1748−52.
9. Hraber P, Kuiken C, Yusim K. Evidence for human leukocyte antigen heterozygote advantage against hepatitis C virus infection. *Hepatology* 2007;**46**:1713−21.
10. van Oosterhout C. A new theory of MHC evolution: beyond selection on the immune genes. *Proc. R. Soc. B* 2009;**276**:657−65. Available from: http://dx.doi.org/10.1098/rspb.2008.1299.
11. Abi-Rached L, Jobin MJ, Kulkarni S, Mcwhinnie A, Dalva K, Gragert L, et al. The shaping of modern human immune systems by multiregional admixture with archaic humans. *Science* 2011;**334**:89−94.
12. Trowsdale J, Knight JC. Major histocompatibility complex genomics and human disease. *Annu Rev Genomics Hum Genet* 2013;**14**:301−23.
13. Apps R, Qi Y, Carlson JM, Chen H, Gao X, Thomas R, et al. Influence of HLA-C expression level on HIV control. *Science* 2013;**340**(6128):87−91.

14. Cohn SK, Weaver LT. The Black Death and AIDS: CCR5-Δ32 in genetics and history. *QJM* 2006;**99**(8):497−503.

15. Lim JK, Louie CY, Glaser C, Jean C, Johnson B, Johnson H, et al. Genetic deficiency of chemokine receptor CCR5 is a strong risk factor for symptomatic West Nile virus infection: a meta-analysis of 4 cohorts in the US epidemic. *J Infect Dis* 2008;**197**(2):262−5.

16. Lim JK, McDermott DH, Lisco A, Foster GA, Krysztof D, Follmann D, et al. CCR5 deficiency is a risk factor for early clinical manifestations of West Nile virus infection but not for viral transmission. *J Infect Dis* 2010;**201**(2):178−85.

17. Kouyuki Hirayasu, et al. Significant association of KIR2DL3-HLA-C1 combination with cerebral malaria and implications for co-evolution of KIR and HLA. *PLoS Pathog* 2012;**8** (3):e1002565.

18. Martin MP, Carrington M. Immunogenetics of HIV disease. *Immunol Rev* 2013;**254** (1):245−64.

19. Hertz T, Oshansky CM, Roddam PL, DeVincenzo JP, Caniza MA, Jojic N, et al. HLA targeting efficiency correlates with human T-cell response magnitude and with mortality from influenza A infection. *Proc Natl Acad Sci USA* 2013;**110**(33):13492−7.

20. Ng MH, Lau KM, Li L, Cheng SH, Chan WY, Hui PK, et al. Association of human-leukocyte-antigen class I (B*0703) and class II (DRB1*0301) genotypes with susceptibility and resistance to the development of severe acute respiratory syndrome. *J Infect Dis* 2004;**190**(3):515−18.

21. Lin M, Tseng HK, Trejaut JA, Lee HL, Loo JH, Chu CC, et al. Association of HLA class I with severe acute respiratory syndrome coronavirus infection. *BMC Med Genet* 2003;**4**:9.

22. Stephens HA. HLA and other gene associations with dengue disease severity. *Curr Top Microbiol Immunol* 2010;**338**:99−114.

23. Pereyra F, et al. The major genetic determinants of HIV-1 control affect HLA class I peptide presentation. *Science* 2010;**330**:1551−7.

24. Hertz T, Nolan D, James I, John M, Gaudieri S, Phillips E, et al. Mapping the landscape of host-pathogen coevolution: HLA class I binding and its relationship with evolutionary conservation in human and viral proteins. *J Virol* 2011;**85**(3):1310−21.

25. de Groot NG, Heijmans CMC, Zoet YM, de Ru AH, Verreck FA, van Veelen PA, et al. AIDS-protective HLA-B*27/B*57 and chimpanzee MHC class I molecules target analogous conserved areas of HIV-1/SIVcpz. *Proc Natl Acad Sci USA* 2010;**107**(34):15175−80.

26. Hoof I, Kesmir C, Lund O, Nielsen M. Humans with chimpanzee-like major histocompatibility complex-specificities control HIV-1 infection. *AIDS* 2008;**12**:1299−303.

27. de Groot NG, Otting N, Doxiadis GG, Balla-Jhagjhoorsingh SS, Heeney JL, van Rood JJ, et al. Evidence for an ancient selective sweep in the MHC class I gene repertoire of chimpanzees. *Proc Natl Acad Sci USA* 2002;**99**(18):11748−53.

28. Poland GA, Ovsyannikova IG, Jacobson RM, Smith DI. Heterogeneity in vaccine immune response: the role of immunogenetics and the emerging field of vaccinomics. *Clin Pharmacol Ther* 2007;**82**(6):653−64.

29. Kennedy RB, Ovsyannika IG, Lambert ND, Haralambieva, Poland G. The personal touch: strategies toward personalized vaccines and predicting immune responses to them. *Expert Rev Vaccines* 2014;**13**(5):657−69.

30. Wang C, Tang J, Song W, et al. HLA and cytokine gene polymorphisms are independently associated with responses to hepatitis B vaccination. *Hepatology* 2004;**39**(4):978−88.

31. Li Y, Ni R, Song W, et al. Clear and independent associations of several HLA-DRB1 alleles with differential antibody responses to hepatitis B vaccination in youth. *Hum Genet* 2009;**126**(5):685−96.

32. Desombere I, Willems A, Leroux-Roels G. Response to hepatitis B vaccine: multiple HLA genes are involved. *Tissue Antigens* 1998;**51**(6):593−604.

33. Hohler T, Stradmann-Bellinghausen B, Starke R, et al. C4A deficiency and nonresponse to hepatitis B vaccination. *J Hepatol* 2002;**37**(3):387−92.

34. De Silvestri A, Pasi A, Martinetti M, et al. Family study of non-responsiveness to hepatitis B vaccine confirms the importance of HLA class III C4A locus. *Genes Immun* 2001;**2**:367−72.

35. Stachowski J, Kramer J, Füst G, Maciejewski J, Baldamus CA, Petrányi GG. Relationship between the reactivity to hepatitis B virus vaccination and the frequency of MHC class I, II and III alleles in haemodialysis patients. *Scand J Immunol* 1995;**42**(1):60−5.

36. Davila S, Froeling FE, Tan A, Bonnard C, Boland GJ, Snippe H, et al. New genetic associations detected in a host response study to hepatitis B vaccine. *Genes Immun* 2010;**11** (3):232−8.

37. Hennig BJ, Fielding K, Broxholme J, Diatta M, Mendy M, et al. Correction: host genetic factors and vaccine-induced immunity to hepatitis B virus infection. *PLoS One* 2011;**6**(2). Available from: http://dx.doi.org/10.1371/journal.pone.0012273.

38. Wu TW, Chen CF, Lai SK, Lin HH, Chu CC, Wang LY. SNP rs7770370 in HLA-DPB1 loci as a major genetic determinant of response to booster hepatitis B vaccination: results of a genome-wide association study. *J Gastroenterol Hepatol* 2015;**30**(5):891−9.

39. Ovsyannikova IG, Pankratz VS, Vierkant RA, et al. Consistency of HLA associations between two independent measles vaccine cohorts: a replication study. *Vaccine* 2012;**30** (12):2146−52.

40. Haralambieva IH, Ovsyannikova IG, Pankratz VS, Kennedy RB, Jacobson RM, Poland GA. The genetic basis for interindividual immune response variation to measles vaccine: new understanding and new vaccine approaches. *Expert Rev Vaccines* 2013;**12**(1):57−70.

41. Dhiman N, Poland GA, Cunningham JM, Jacobson RM, Ovsyannikova IG, Vierkant RA, et al. Variations in measles vaccine-specific humoral immunity by polymorphisms in SLAM and CD46 measles virus receptors. *J Allergy Clin Immunol* 2007;**120**(3):666−72.

42. Ovsyannikova IG, Haralambieva IH, Vierkant RA, et al. The association of CD46, SLAM, and CD209 cellular receptor gene SNPs with variations in measles vaccine-induced immune responses: a replication study and examination of novel polymorphisms. *Hum Hered* 2011;**72**(3):206−23.

43. Clifford HD, Hayden CM, Khoo SK, Zhang G, Le Souëf PN, Richmond P. CD46 measles virus receptor polymorphisms influence receptor protein expression and primary measles vaccine responses in naive Australian children. *Clin Vaccine Immunol* 2012;**19**(5):704−10.

44. Dhiman N, Ovsyannikova IG, Cunningham JM, Vierkant RA, Kennedy RB, Pankratz VS, et al. Associations between measles vaccine immunity and single-nucleotide polymorphisms in cytokine and cytokine receptor genes. *J Infect Dis* 2007;**195**(1):21−9.

45. Haralambieva IH, Ovsyannikova IG, Kennedy RB, Vierkant RA, Pankratz VS, Jacobson RM, et al. Associations between single nucleotide polymorphisms and haplotypes in cytokine and cytokine receptor genes and immunity to measles vaccination. *Vaccine* 2011;**29** (45):7883−95.

46. White SJ, Haralambieva IH, Ovsyannikova IG, Vierkant RA, O'Byrne MM, Poland GA. Replication of associations between cytokine and cytokine receptor single nucleotide polymorphisms and measles-specific adaptive immunophenotypic extremes. *Hum Immunol* 2012;**73**(6):636−40.

47. Ovsyannikova IG, Pankratz VS, Larrabee BR, Jacobson RM, Poland GA. HLA genotypes and rubella vaccine immune response: additional evidence. *Vaccine* 2014;**32**(33):4206−13.

48. Lambert ND, Haralambieva IH, Kennedy RB, Ovsyannikova IG, Pankratz VS, Poland GA. Polymorphisms in HLA-DPB1 are associated with differences in rubella virus-specific humoral immunity after vaccination. *J Infect Dis* 2015;**211**(6):898−905.

49. Ovsyannikova IG, Pankratz VS, Salk HM, Kennedy RB, Poland GA. HLA alleles associated with the adaptive immune response to smallpox vaccine: a replication study. *Hum Genet* 2014;**133**(9):1083−92.

50. Gartland AJ, Li S, McNevin J, Tomaras GD, Gottardo R, Janes H, et al. Analysis of HLA A*02 association with vaccine efficacy in the RV144 HIV-1 vaccine trial. *J Virol* 2014;**88** (15):8242−55.

51. Uzicanin A, Zimmerman L. Field effectiveness of live attenuated measles-containing vaccines: a review of published literature. *J Infect Dis* 2011;**204**(Suppl. 1):S133−48.

52. De Serres G, Boulianne N, Defay F, Brousseau N, Benoît M, Lacoursière S, et al. Higher risk of measles when the first dose of a 2-dose schedule of measles vaccine is given at 12−14 months versus 15 months of age. *Clin Infect Dis* 2012;**55**(3):394−402.

53. Hirano A, Kurita-Taniguchi M, Katayama Y, Matsumoto M, Wong TC, Seya T. Ligation of human CD46 with purified complement C3b or F(ab')(2) of monoclonal antibodies enhances isoform-specific interferon gamma-dependent nitric oxide production in macrophages. *J Biochem* 2002;**132**(1):83−91.

54. Ovsyannikova IG, Haralambieva IH, Kennedy RB, O'Byrne MM, Pankratz VS, Poland GA. Genetic variation in IL18R1 and IL18 genes and inteferon γ ELISPOT response to smallpox vaccination: an unexpected relationship. *J Infect Dis* 2013;**208**(9):1422−30. http://dx.doi.org/10.1093/infdis/jit341.

55. Mudd PA, Ericsen AJ, Walsh AD, Leon EJ, Wilson NA, Maness NJ, et al. CD8 + T cell escape mutations in simian immunodeficiency virus SIVmac239 cause fitness defects in vivo, and many revert after transmission. *J Virol* 2011;**85**:12804−10.

56. Schneidewind A, Brockman MA, Yang R, Adam RI, Li B, Le Gall S, et al. Escape from the dominant HLA-B27-restricted cytotoxic T-lymphocyte response in Gag is associated with a dramatic reduction in human immunodeficiency virus type 1 replication. *J Virol* 2007;**81**(22):12382−93.

57. Brockman MA, Schneidewind A, Lahaie M, Schmidt A, Miura T, Desouza I, et al. Escape and compensation from early HLA-B57-mediated cytotoxic T-lymphocyte pressure on human immunodeficiency virus type 1 Gag alter capsid interactions with cyclophilin A. *J Virol* 2007;**81**(22):12608−18.

58. Fellay J, Frahm N, Shianna KV, Cirulli ET, Casimiro DR, Robertson MN, et al. Host genetic determinants of T cell responses to the MRKAd5 HIV-1 gag/pol/nef vaccine in the step trial. *J Infect Dis* 2011;**203**(6):773−9.

59. Fellay J, et al. A whole-genome association study of major determinants for host control of HIV-1. *Science* 2007;**317**:944−7.

60. Dalmasso C, et al. Distinct genetic loci control plasma HIV-RNA and cellular HIV-DNA levels in HIV-1 infection: the ANRS Genome Wide Association 01 study. *PLoS One* 2008;**3**:e3907.

61. Fellay J, et al. Common genetic variation and the control of HIV-1 in humans. *PLoS Genet* 2009;**5**:e1000791.

62. Thomas R, et al. HLA-C cell surface expression and control of HIV/AIDS correlate with a variant upstream of HLA-C. *Nat Genet* 2009;**41**:1290−4.

63. Kulkarni S, et al. Differential microRNA regulation of HLA-C expression and its association with HIV control. *Nature* 2011;**472**:495−8.

64. Blais ME, et al. High frequency of HIV mutations associated with HLA-C suggests enhanced HLA-C-restricted CTL selective pressure associated with an AIDS-protective polymorphism. *J Immunol* 2012;**188**:4663−70.

65. Rolland M, Nickle DC, Deng W, Frahm N, Brander C, Learn GH, et al. Recognition of HIV-1 peptides by host CTL is related to HIV-1 similarity to human proteins. *PLoS One* 2007;**2**(9):e823.

66. Kosmrlj A, et al. Effects of thymic selection of the T-cell repertoire on HLA class I-associated control of HIV infection. *Nature* 2010;**465**:350−4.

67. Kløverpris HN, McGregor R, McLaren JE, Ladell K, Harndahl M, Stryhn A, et al. Bias and immunodominance in HIV-1 infection. *J Immunol* 2015;**194**(11):5329−45.

68. Chen H, Ndhlovu ZM, Liu D, Porter LC, Fang JW, Darko S, et al. TCR clonotypes modulate the protective effect of HLA class I molecules in HIV-1 infection. *Nat Immunol* 2012;**13**:691−700.

69. Jonathan WY. Confronting complexity: review real-world immunodominance in antiviral CD8 + T cell responses. *Immunity* 2006;**25**:533−43.

70. Hartman IZ, Kim A, Cotter RJ, Walter K, Dalai SK, Boronina T, et al. A reductionist cell-free major histocompatibility complex class II antigen processing system identifies immunodominant epitopes. *Nat Med* 2010;**16**(11):1333−40.

71. Hughes AL, Hughes MK. Self peptides bound by HLA class I molecules are derived from highly conserved regions of a set of evolutionarily conserved proteins. *Immunogenetics* 1995;**41**(5):257−62.

72. Verweij MC, Horst D, Griffin BD, Luteijn RD, Davison AJ, et al. Viral inhibition of the transporter associated with antigen processing (TAP): a striking example of functional convergent evolution. *PLoS Pathog* 2015;**11**(4):e1004743.

73. Almeida CA, Bronke C, Roberts SG, McKinnon E, Keane NM, Chopra A, et al. Translation of HLA-HIV associations to the cellular level: HIV adapts to inflate CD8 T cell responses against Nef and HLA-adapted variant epitopes. *J Immunol* 2011;**187**(5):2502−13.

74. Keane NM, Roberts SG, Almeida CA, Krishnan T, Chopra A, Demaine E, et al. High-avidity, high-IFNγ-producing CD8 T-cell responses following immune selection during HIV-1 infection. *Immunol Cell Biol* 2012;**90**(2):224−34.

75. Karlsson AC, Iversen AK, Chapman JM, de Oliviera T, Spotts G, McMichael AJ, et al. Sequential broadening of CTL responses in early HIV-1 infection is associated with viral escape. *PLoS One* 2007;**2**(2):e225.

76. Carrington M, Martin MP, van Bergen J. KIR-HLA intercourse in HIV disease. *Trends Microbiol* 2008;**16**:620−7.

77. Alter G, Heckerman D, Schneidewind A, Fadda L, Kadie CM, Carlson JM, et al. HIV-1 adaptation to NK-cell-mediated immune pressure. *Nature* 2011;**476**:96−100.

78. Huang J, et al. HLA-B*35-Px-mediated acceleration of HIV-1 infection by increased inhibitory immunoregulatory impulses. *J Exp Med* 2009;**206**:2959−66.

79. Lipsitch M, O'Hagan JJ. Patterns of antigenic diversity and the mechanisms that maintain them. *J R Soc Interface* 2007;**4**:787−802.

80. McMicheal AJ, Phillips RE. Escape of human immunodeficiency virus from immune control. *Annu Rev Immunol* 1997;**15**:271−96.

81. Goulder PJ, Walker BD. HIV and HLA class I: an evolving relationship. *Immunity* 2012;**37**(3):126 40.

82. Moore CB, John M, James IR, Christiansen FT, Witt CS, Mallal SA. Evidence of HIV-1 adaptation to HLA-restricted immune responses at a population level. *Science* 2002;**296** (5572):1439–43.

83. Carlson JM, Le AQ, Shahid A, Brumme ZL. HIV-1 adaptation to HLA: a window into virus-host immune interactions. *Trends Microbiol* 2015;**23**(4):212–24.

84. Leslie A, Price DA, Mkhize P, Bishop K, Rathod A, Day C, et al. Differential selection pressure exerted on HIV by CTL targeting identical epitopes but restricted by distinct HLA alleles from the same HLA supertype. *J Immunol* 2006;**177**(7):4699–708.

85. John M, Heckerman D, James I, Park LP, Carlson JM, Chopra A, et al. Adaptive interactions between HLA and HIV-1: highly divergent selection imposed by HLA class I molecules with common supertype motifs. *J Immunol* 2010;**184**(8):4368–77.

86. Dong T, Zhang Y, Xu KY, Yan H, James I, Peng Y, et al. Extensive HLA-driven viral diversity following a narrow-source HIV-1 outbreak in rural China. *Blood* 2011;**118** (1):98–106.

87. Lai-Goldman M, Faruki H. Abacavir hypersensitivity: a model system for pharmacogenetic test adoption. *Genet Med* 2008;**10**:874–8.

88. Mallal S, Nolan D, Witt C, Masel G, Martin AM, Moore C, et al. Association between presence of HLA-B*5701, HLA-DR7, and HLA-DQ3 and hypersensitivity to HIV-1 reverse-transcriptase inhibitor abacavir. *Lancet* 2002;**359**(9308):727–32.

89. Mallal S, Phillips E, Carosi G, Molina JM, Workman C, Tomazic J, et al. HLA-B*5701 screening for hypersensitivity to abacavir. *N Engl J Med* 2008;**358**(6):568–79.

90. Saag M, Balu R, Phillips E, Brachman P, Martorell C, Burman W, et al. Study of hypersensitivity to abacavir and pharmacogenetic evaluation study team. High sensitivity of human leukocyte antigen-b*5701 as a marker for immunologically confirmed abacavir hypersensitivity in white and black patients. *Clin Infect Dis* 2008;**46**(7):1111–18.

91. Pulendran B, Li S, Nakaya HI. Systems vaccinology. *Immunity* 2010;**33**(4):516–29.

92. Yang OO, Ali A, Kasahara N, Faure-Kumar E, Bae JY, Picker LJ, et al. Short conserved sequences of HIV-1 are highly immunogenic and shift immunodominance. *J Virol* 2015;**89** (2):1195–204.

Part IV

Advanced Vaccine Development

Chapter 7

Methodical Considerations

P.B. Gilbert[1,2] and R. Gottardo[1,2]

[1]*Fred Hutchinson Cancer Research Center, Seattle, WA, United States,* [2]*University of Washington, Seattle, WA, United States*

In this chapter, we discuss statistical issues for assessing vaccine efficacy and for assessing and developing immune correlates of vaccine efficacy. We begin by comparing and contrasting concepts and measures of vaccine efficacy that have been used. Then, for the rest of the chapter, we focus on assessing unconditional cumulative vaccine efficacy for susceptibility over time and correlates of that efficacy based on individual randomized preventive vaccine efficacy trials. After presenting a general integrated framework for assessing how vaccine efficacy depends on immune response markers and on genotypic/phenotypic features of exposing pathogens, we describe some major statistical challenges posed to this problem and sketch approaches to addressing these challenges.

INTRODUCTION TO VACCINE EFFICACY

Several measures of vaccine efficacy (VE) are of interest for vaccine evaluation.[1,2] One class of VE parameters measures direct benefits of vaccination based on randomization of individuals to receive the candidate vaccine or placebo, including "VE for susceptibility" (VE$_S$). VE$_S$ measures the degree to which vaccine recipients have reduced risk of acquiring clinically significant infection with the pathogen under study compared to placebo recipients. "VE for progression" and "VE for infectiousness" are two other direct effect parameters, measuring in individuals who acquire pathogen infection the degree to which vaccination slows disease progression and lowers the risk of secondary transmission, respectively.[3] Another class of VE parameters measure indirect or aggregate (direct + indirect) benefits of vaccination to groups of individuals based on cluster randomized trials (CRTs) that randomize groups to receive the candidate vaccine or a control condition. A parallel CRT design randomizes groups/clusters (e.g., villages) to receive vaccine

Human Vaccines: Emerging Technologies in Design and Development.
DOI: http://dx.doi.org/10.1016/B978-0-12-802302-0.00006-6

or control, and vaccinates all individuals (or as many as possible) within the clusters assigned vaccine. "Total VE" compares the risk of clinically significant infection between vaccinated and control clusters and assesses the aggregate of the direct benefit of the vaccine to reduce susceptibility and the indirect benefit to reduce the amount of pathogen exposure via reducing the pool of pathogen infected individuals (herd immunity). In addition, a double-layered randomization design randomizes clusters to vaccine or control, and, within clusters assigned vaccine, randomizes individuals to vaccine versus placebo. These designs enable estimation of "Indirect VE" that isolates the herd immunity benefit of vaccination.[2]

While most CRTs have used parallel group designs where each cluster receives vaccine or a control condition throughout the study, increasingly one-way cross-over "stepped wedge" designs are being used in which every cluster eventually receives vaccine and the order of vaccine initiation is randomized.[4–10] Stepped wedge designs have two main advantages over parallel group designs: firstly they can be more acceptable ethically by avoiding pure control groups, which is especially important for vaccines with prior evidence of vaccine efficacy and secondly their implementation may be logistically simpler by incrementally rolling out a vaccination campaign to different clusters. However, stepped wedge designs are usually less statistically efficient than parallel group designs, and it is more difficult to achieve unbiased estimation of VE.[11]

Another distinction among VE parameters is between "vaccine efficacy" and "vaccine effectiveness." Vaccine efficacy parameters are designed to capture direct biological benefit of the vaccine,[12] and prioritize achieving internal validity through rigorous experimental control of bias via randomization and double-blinding. VE_S is the pre-dominant parameter for measuring vaccine efficacy, typically being the central measure used by the Food and Drug Administration and other regulatory authorities.[13] Vaccine effectiveness, distinct from vaccine efficacy, is designed to capture the net effectiveness of a vaccination program accounting for behavioral and ecological factors, under more natural field conditions, and prioritize achieving results that inform real-world public health impact.[13,14] Vaccine effectiveness may be assessed by randomized trials (individual or cluster) with nonplacebo control groups, rendering comparisons of endpoint rates informative about the aggregate impact of biological and behavioral effects of a vaccination program.[12,15] It also may be assessed in non-randomized Phase IV postlicensure studies, with epidemiological analysis methods needed to estimate public health impact (e.g., with the case test-negative design).[16] In the lifecycle of vaccine development, in the period before the first highly efficacious vaccine is identified, research typically centers on vaccine efficacy and on VE_S in particular, and, after one or more vaccines are licensed, more attention is turned toward vaccine effectiveness. Tracking this pattern, individual randomized trials predominate for Phase 2b intermediate-sized vaccine efficacy trials[17–20] and Phase 3 licensure trials, with cluster randomized trials becoming more important for Phase 3 and 4 trials.

Given the theme of this book to generate and leverage modern technologies to accelerate development and improvement of vaccines against the toughest pathogens for which highly efficacious vaccines do not yet exist, henceforth we focus on the assessment of VE_S based on individual-randomized placebo controlled Phase 2b or 3 efficacy trials. For simplicity we refer to VE_S as VE. Generally vaccine efficacy trials have used symptomatic disease as the study endpoint for VE, i.e., clinically significant infection,[21] or just infection for settings where infection is a validated surrogate endpoint for a disease endpoint (e.g., HIV infection is a validated surrogate endpoint for AIDS). Recently infection endpoint trials have been initiated for settings where infection has not yet been validated as a surrogate endpoint; such trials rapidly screen candidate vaccines using the unproven putative surrogate for selection into Phase 3 disease endpoint trials (e.g., TB vaccines[22]). We refer to the study endpoint for measuring VE as clinically significant infection.

PRIMARY OBJECTIVE TO ASSESS VE FOR SUSCEPTIBILITY IN INDIVIDUAL RANDOMIZED PREVENTIVE VACCINE EFFICACY TRIALS

Several different VE for susceptibility parameters have been used. We discuss major distinctions in these parameters in two dimensions, first whether they condition on measured exposure to the pathogen and second whether they express the instantaneous or cumulative incidence of the study endpoint.

Exposure-Conditional VE vs Unconditional VE

Exposure-conditional VE measures a vaccine vs placebo contrast in the probability a susceptible individual experiences the endpoint conditional on data documenting that the individual was exposed or potentially exposed to the pathogen. For example, the measured exposure could be bites from malaria infected mosquitos in a challenge trial,[23-25] membership in a household with a family member documented to be infected with the pathogen,[26] or membership in a sexual partnership with an individual documented to be infected.[26-30] Unconditional VE measures a contrast in the probability (risk) of acquiring the endpoint over a specified time period without conditioning on individual exposure data.[31] Exposure-conditional VE is generally preferred where feasible for its interpretation as direct biological reduction in susceptibility to acquiring the study endpoint and because it can be estimated with greater statistical precision.[32] Moreover, exposure-conditional VE is advantageous for sieve analysis (discussed below) by allowing incorporation of genotypic/phenotypic data about the exposing pathogens that are unavailable for unconditional VE. Therefore, an important area of research is development of data collection designs and tools that directly document pathogen exposure[33,34]; e.g., the HIV Vaccine Trials

Network is currently studying the sensitivity and specificity of HIV specific PCR on self-administered daily vaginal swabs to detect HIV in semen. The accuracy of the exposure data determines whether conditional VE may be reliably used—affirmative if specificity and sensitivity of exposure diagnosis is high, in which case a validation set statistical method[34] or measurement error statistical method[35,36] may be used. If specificity or sensitivity is low, however, then even the most advanced statistical methods are unable to provide reliable estimates of exposure-conditional VE, tipping the argument in favor of using unconditional VE parameters. Even if unconditional VE is used, designing the inclusion/exclusion criteria to minimize the number of trial participants that are never exposed to the pathogen can improve resource efficiency.[37] In designing a particular efficacy trial, simulation studies comparing exposure-conditional and unconditional VE methods may be used to select the most suitable approach.

Generally, special structures in the pathogen exposure/acquisition process and in opportunities to measure this process have been required to support the exposure-conditional approach, including challenge studies, household studies, and partners studies as noted above. For sexually acquired infections, in principle the discordant partners studies (with one member infected with the pathogen and the other member uninfected) would effectively enable the approach; however, to our knowledge these designs have not yet been used for preventive vaccines. Most vaccine efficacy trials have used unconditional VE, including all HIV trials. Use of exposure-conditional VE is illustrated by pertussis vaccine trials.[38] A research objective is development of automatic electronic measurement technology[39] or other technology (e.g., self-report risk-behavior data collection via mobile technology) that improves diagnostic quality to the point of warranting use of exposure-conditional VE in more vaccine trials.

Instantaneous VE vs Cumulative VE

Given that most vaccine efficacy trials use unconditional VE for susceptibility parameters, henceforth we restrict attention to these parameters. Two major such parameters are based on instantaneous incidence and cumulative incidence of the endpoint.[40] Instantaneous VE may be measured by one minus the ratio (vaccine group/placebo group) of instantaneous incidence rates (i.e., hazards) over a specified follow-up period, whereas cumulative VE may be measured by one minus the ratio (vaccine/placebo) of cumulative incidence rates up to a specified time point after randomization. Typically a proportional hazards model is used to estimate instantaneous VE, which assumes that VE is the same over all follow-up time, i.e., that efficacy does not wane distal from receipt of the immunizations. Cumulative VE may be estimated by separately estimating the probability of the endpoint in the vaccine and placebo group (e.g., with the Kaplan-Meier method), making no assumptions about whether and how VE changes over time.

Statistical Science Philosophy for the Assessment of VE

The following principles may guide selection of the VE parameter and the analytic approach for estimating VE in the primary efficacy analysis, which also apply for the assessment of immune correlates of VE considered next.

1. Select a VE parameter that is interpretable for the primary scientific objective.
2. List all assumptions needed for the selected method to provide a valid (unbiased) estimate of the VE parameter. Favor methods that only require assumptions that are known to be true or that can be well tested based on internal and/or external data.
3. If the selected method uses an assumption that is very likely false and not fully verifiable from data, determine the sensitivity of the method to violations of the assumption. If the method is known to be robust, then its use may be justified as an approximately valid method. Otherwise, avoid using the method. If it is nonetheless used, include in the results a sensitivity analysis showing how estimates of VE vary with violations of the assumption.
4. Favor methods that use all information in the collected data and in the known-true assumptions, to maximize statistical efficiency.

Based on these principles, the cumulative VE parameter may often be the most principled choice. Firstly, it is simple to interpret, as the percent multiplicative reduction in the probability of acquiring the endpoint through time t in follow-up, Risk(t), and it measures a causal effect of assignment to vaccine versus placebo. Secondly, it can be estimated without any assumptions about how VE changes over time, which is usually relevant given the potential for waning VE and the explicit objective in trials to study how VE changes over time. Furthermore, it can be estimated without assuming anything about the amount of heterogeneity of HIV risk, as Risk(t) is equivalently the average probability of endpoint occurrence over all subpopulations in the study population. Thirdly, statistical methods are available for estimating cumulative VE that account for all of the collected baseline covariate data, maximizing efficiency by leveraging information in covariates prognostic for the endpoint and for VE without requiring correct modeling of these associations; moreover these methods can correct for nonrandom dropout by modeling the association of dropout with participant covariates.[41–43]

We contrast the cumulative VE approach to the standard approach that has been used for many primary analyses—assessment of instantaneous VE via a Cox proportional hazards model. Under the proportional hazards assumption, instantaneous VE measures a causal effect of assignment to vaccine versus placebo and has clear interpretation as the percent multiplicative reduction (vaccine vs placebo) in the incidence of the endpoint during a short interval of follow-up. However, if the proportional hazards assumption fails, then the instantaneous VE parameter does not measure a causal effect of vaccination[44] and becomes difficult to interpret, because it depends on the distribution of drop-out.[45] Moreover, heterogeneity in risk of the study endpoint can cause bias in the estimation of the hazard ratio.[37] In addition, standard covariate-adjusted analyses of instantaneous VE achieved by fitting Cox regression models do not estimate the instantaneous VE parameter of interest, and the validity of estimation requires a correctly specified Cox model that will often be mis-specified due to lack of knowledge. Therefore, we judge the cumulative VE parameter to more closely adhere to the principles listed above. Nevertheless, in practice instantaneous VE has often served as a reasonable approximation to VE averaged over follow-up time, and is approximately valid for efficacy trials where vaccine efficacy is approximately constant over time. We encourage greater consideration of the cumulative VE approach, and henceforth focus on this approach.

CUMULATIVE VE UNIFIED FRAMEWORK FOR OVERALL VE AND IMMUNE CORRELATES OF VE

Table 7.1 shows cumulative VE parameters that can be used as a basis for assessment of overall vaccine efficacy, vaccine efficacy in participant subgroups defined by baseline covariates, vaccine efficacy in participant subgroups defined by measured immune responses to vaccination, and vaccine efficacy against particular genotypes or phenotypes of the pathogen. Collectively these objectives may be referred to as assessing vaccine efficacy and assessing immune correlates of VE, where "immune correlates" entails integrated assessment of how VE depends on vaccine-induced immune responses and on features of the pathogen. In Table 7.1, the notation X denotes baseline participant characteristics such as sex, age, geographic region, nutrition, host immune genetic factors such as major histocompatibility types, seropositivity to the pathogen, or high-dimensional measurements of the microbiome.

In Table 7.1, the notation S denotes an immune response (IR) marker, which is a measured immune response to vaccination with measurement taken either at a fixed visit time τ shortly after part or all of the immunization series (typically 2−4 weeks post), or at a series of time points during follow-up. The IR marker S may be a single variable such as neutralization titer to a particular strain of the pathogen inside or outside the vaccine construct. Alternatively, S may be high-dimensional such as the full set of readouts of the T or B cell repertoire or of binding antibody responses to linear peptides tiled over a surface protein measured by peptide micro-array[47−49] (see chapter: Systems Vaccinology). The notation J denotes a genotypic or phenotypic feature of the pathogen at the time of exposure, with "genotype" referring to any feature defined by the nucleotides or amino acids of the pathogen determined by sequencing (e.g., Sanger

TABLE 7.1 For a Randomized Placebo-Controlled Preventive Vaccine Efficacy (VE) Parameters for Quantifying Reduction in Susceptibility Efficacy for Susceptibility (VE) Parameters for Quantifying Reduction in Susceptibility to Acquire the Primary Endpoint (Clinically Significant Infection)

Symbol	Name	Meaning	Objectives
Overall Vaccine Efficacy			
Vrisk(t) Prisk(t)	Cumulative risk/attack rate of the endpoint for the Vx or Plc group	Expected probability a vaccinee experiences at the endpoint by time t^a	Input for VE(t)
VE(t)	Overall vaccine efficacy VE(t) = 1 − Vrisk(t)/Prisk(t)	Percent reduction (V vs P) in cumulative risk of the endpoint by time t	Primary objective to assess overall VE by a specified late time-point t Secondary objective: VE over time
Baseline Subgroup Vaccine Efficacy ($X = x$ denotes a specific subgroup defined by baseline covariates)			
Vrisk(t|x) Prisk(t|x)	Baseline subgroup cumul. risk for Vx, Plc	Same as Vrisk(t), Prisk(t) in the subgroup with $X = x$	Input for VE(t|x)
VE(t|x)	Baseline subgroup VE: VE(t|x) = 1 − Vrisk(t|x)/Prisk(t|x)	Same as VE(t) in the baseline subgroup with $X = x$	Secondary objective to assess differential VE by baseline subgroup (effect modification)
Immune Response (IR) Marker Subgroup Vaccine Efficacy ($S = s$ denotes a specific subgroup defined by the readout(s) of one or more immune responses to vaccination measured at a fixed time τ or serially)			
Vrisk(t|s) Prisk(t|s)	IR marker subgroup cumulative risk for Vx	Same as Vrisk(t), Prisk(t) in the subgroup with $S = s^b$	Input for VE(t|s)
VE(t|s)	IR marker subgroup VE: VE(t|s) = 1 − Vrisk(t|s)/Prisk(t|s)	Same as VE(t) in the subgroup with $S = s$	Secondary objective to assess differential VE(t) by IR marker subgroup (immune CoPs)

(Continued)

TABLE 7.1 (Continued)

Symbol	Name	Meaning	Objectives
Baseline x Immune Response (IR) Marker Subgroup Vaccine Efficacy ($(X = x, S = s)$ a specific subgroup)			
Vrisk$(t|s,x)$ Prisk$(t|s,x)$	Baseline x IR marker subgroup cumulative risk for Vx, Plc	Same as Vrisk(t), Prisk(t) in the subgroup with $X = x$, $S = s$	Input for VE$(t|s,x)$
VE$(t|s,x)$	Baseline x IR marker subgroup VE: VE$(t|s,x)$ = 1-Vrisk$(t|s,x)$/Prisk$(t|s,x)$	Same as VE(t) in the subgroup with $X = x$ and $S = s$	Exploratory objective to assess differential immune CoPs by baseline subgroup (immune CoP effect modification)
Baseline x Immune Response (IR) Marker Subgroup Pathogen Type-Specific Vaccine Efficacy			
Vrisk$(t,j|s,x)$ Prisk$(t,j|s,x)$	Baseline x IR marker subgroup type j cumul. risk for Vx, Plc	Same as Vrisk$(t|s,x)$, Prisk$(t|s,x)$ for the pathogen type j endpoint	Input for VE$(t,j|s,x)$
VE$(t,j|s,x)$	Baseline x IR marker subgroup type j VE: VE$(t,j|s,x)$ = $1 - $Vrisk$(t,j|s,x)$/ Prisk$(t,j|s,x)$	Same as VE$(t|s,x)$ against the pathogen type j endpoint	Exploratory objective to assess differential type j immune CoPs by baseline subgroup (immune CoP effect modification)

[a]The time origin for endpoint assessment is the date of randomization/first immunization for the modified intention-to-treat (MITT) analysis and a specified time τ after the immunization series for the per-protocol analysis.

[b]Membership in the subgroup also includes that the vaccinee did not experience the endpoint by the time that the IR marker was measured and would also not have experienced the endpoint had s/he been assigned placebo.[46]

sequencing or next-generation sequencing) and "phenotype" referring to any pathogen feature determined by a biological assay, e.g., a measure of the sensitivity of the pathogen to neutralization by sera from vaccine recipients.[50–52] J may also be a single variable such as the status of whether the pathogen is matched to the vaccine at a given amino acid position or whether the pathogen is of a particular serotype, or it may be high-dimensional such as the full set of data obtained from deep sequencing of the whole genome of the pathogen, constituting hundreds of thousands of data points. The purpose of Table 7.1 is to define a framework for integrated analysis of vaccine efficacy and immune correlates, which is of general interest for arbitrary variables (X, S, V). ... With the development of modern measurement technologies that constitute a thematic topic of this book, these variables are increasingly high-dimensional, providing opportunities for enriched understanding of the factors affecting VE and posing challenges to data processing and analysis.

In the notation of Table 7.1, variables to the right of the conditioning symbol | indicate the participant subgroup for which vaccine efficacy is assessed, which is either the whole study cohort (no variables), a baseline subgroup (X), an IR marker subgroup (S), or a subgroup defined by both X and S. The objective to assess immune correlates of VE can be defined as estimation and testing of VE in subgroups defined by S and by (X, S), both for all pathogen types $(VE(t|S), VE(t|S,X))$ and for specific pathogen types $(VE(t_j|S), VE(t_j|S, X))$. All of the VE parameters in Table 7.1 have interpretation as the multiplicative reduction (vaccine vs placebo) in the average probability of the endpoint by time t, averaging over all baseline characteristics represented in the study population, measured or unmeasured. As such, the VE parameters average endpoint risks over unmeasured factors related to pathogen exposure or pathogen susceptibility. Even the parameter involving the most data, $VE(t_j|S,X)$, is an average—of type j endpoint risks in the (S, X) subgroup averaged over all baseline characteristics not captured by S and X.

The crucial assumption for reliably learning about all of the VE parameters is random assignment to vaccine or placebo, which guarantees that the two groups being compared have the same distribution of measured and unmeasured predictors of the study endpoint. This implies that the VE parameter measures a causal effect to assignment to vaccine or placebo, isolating the cause and assuring that the effect is not due to any other factor. The two other main assumptions are "no interference"—that the treatment assignment of an individual does not affect the risk of the endpoint for other individuals, and "random censoring"—that participants who drop out have the same risk of the endpoint as participants who do not drop out. Recent advances provide statistical methods for estimating VE without requiring the no interference assumption, based on doubly layered randomized designs mentioned in the introduction.[53,54] In addition, recent advances provide methods for assessing VE relaxing the random censoring assumption.[42,43]

PRIMARY OBJECTIVE: ASSESSMENT OF OVERALL CUMULATIVE VACCINE EFFICACY

The top three panels of Table 7.1 define a cumulative VE parameter that may be used for the primary efficacy analysis. This analysis estimates $VE(t)$ by a fixed follow-up time point such as $t = 2$ years after randomization/enrollment or $t = 2$ years after immune responses are measured at time τ for assessing immune correlates. A typical approach to selecting the sample size of the trial takes the following steps.

1. Select the null hypothesis for vaccine efficacy. For a Phase 2b design the null is zero vaccine efficacy, H_0: $VE(t) \leq 0\%$, and for a Phase 3 design the null is low positive vaccine efficacy, e.g., H_0: $VE(t) \leq 25\%$.[17] Select the type I error rate, typically 1-sided 0.025, and perhaps larger for a Phase 2b design to allow greater power.

2. Determine the fixed t and the "design alternative" fixed level of cumulative vaccine efficacy, $VE_a(t)$, such that the trial must have high power to reject H_0 if $VE(t) = VE_a(t)$ (e.g., specify 90% power). The value $VE_a(t)$ is selected such that if the trial just barely rejects H_0, then a milestone is achieved guiding next steps for the vaccine. If the trial is a Phase 3 trial, this milestone may be a minimal level of efficacy such that mathematical models (and discussions with regulatory authorities) indicate enough public health utility to justify licensure of the vaccine (e.g., $VE_a(t = 2$ years$) = 50\%$). If the trial is an intermediate-sized Phase 2b efficacy trial, this milestone may be enough efficacy to support an immune correlates of VE analysis and to motivate a follow-up Phase 3 trial of a refined version of the vaccine (e.g., $VE_a(t = 1.5$ years$) = 40\%$).

3. Develop an interim monitoring plan for the analysis of $VE(t)$ at a sequence of calendar intervals. The interim analysis results are confidentially reported to the Data Safety Monitoring Board (DSMB) that is charged with protecting the safety of study participants and the scientific integrity of the trial.[55] This sequential monitoring plan typically includes monitoring for potential vaccine harm (evidence for $VE(t) < 0$) and for efficacy futility (evidence that the design alternative $VE(t) \geq VE_a(t)$ can be ruled out with high probability), and may also monitor for very high $VE(t)$ that may indicate an ethical rationale to rapidly make the results public and offer the vaccine to placebo recipients in the trial.[56,57]

4. Specify assumptions about the incidence of the primary endpoint in the placebo group through to time t and about the rate of dropout over time.

5. Based on thousands of simulated trials with $VE(t)$ set to the value of the design alternative $VE_a(t)$, select the sample size to meet all of the above requirements, where for each trial the sequential monitoring plan is performed and the result is tallied as "meeting the design alternative" if, in the presence of the monitoring, the conclusion of the trial is rejection of H_0.

A major design decision is whether to assess VE in the modified intention-to-treat (MITT) cohort or the per-protocol cohort,[58,59] where the MITT cohort is all randomized participants documented to meet key inclusion criteria at baseline (e.g., HIV-uninfected at baseline) and the per-protocol cohort is the subset of randomized participants who received all planned immunizations and meet protocol criteria regarding receipt of the planned immunizations within visit windows. The main advantages of the MITT analysis include: (1) the intention-to-treat analysis is valid based on randomization of treatment assignments, guaranteeing that VE(t) measures a causal effect of assignment to vaccine or placebo; (2) the analysis is closer to "real-world" than the per-protocol analysis by including all participants in the analysis, thus factoring in the impact of some missing immunizations; and (3) the number of study endpoints included in the analysis is greater than for the per-protocol analysis, which can provide greater statistical power (e.g., there were 578 MITT and 250 per-protocol primary dengue disease endpoints in a recent Phase 3 trial[60]). A main advantage of the per-protocol analysis is maximizing the opportunity for maximal VE by restricting to the subgroup most likely to receive the full benefit of the vaccine regimen as designed, which in some settings will make the per-protocol analysis have greater statistical power. In general both analyses are insightful and complementary, such that both are recommended for routine practice[58] and the sample size calculations should consider both analyses; we tend to favor the MITT analysis for the primary analysis given the advantages listed above. The per-protocol analysis may be biased by an imbalance of predictors of the study endpoint between the treatment groups that may arise due to early VE, early differences in dropout, or early differences in immunization-receipt. This fact motivates application of statistical methods designed to correct the bias (e.g., Ref. 41) and of sensitivity analysis methods[61] that assess the robustness of estimates of VE(t) to departures from un-verifiable assumptions that are made by bias-correction methods. Fig. 7.1A illustrates estimation of VE(t) for the MITT analysis of the RV144 HIV vaccine efficacy trial.

STATISTICAL ISSUES IN ASSESSING IMMUNE CORRELATES OF VE VIA ESTIMATION OF VE($t\,|\,s$) OR VE($t\,|\,s,x$)

Development of the Immune Response Markers S

Given the large number of immunological assays and associated component immunological variables that could potentially be evaluated as immune correlates of VE, it is advantageous to first conduct pilot studies to down-select assays into the case-control study.[62] These pilot studies may be conducted during the efficacy trial, or may be based on previous Phase 1/2 trials if the study population is approximately the same as the efficacy trial population. Within an efficacy trial, such pilot studies perform each candidate assay

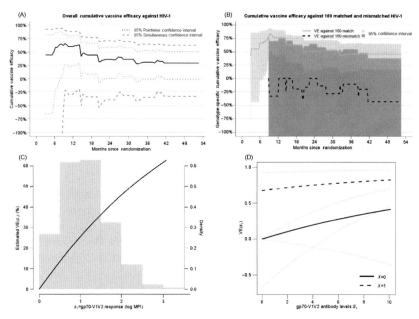

FIGURE 7.1 Illustration of the analysis of overall VE(t) and immune correlates of protection for the RV144 preventive HIV vaccine efficacy trial. (A) Point and 95% confidence interval (CI) estimates of cumulative VE over time since randomization, VE(t) = 1 − Vrisk(t)/Prisk(t); (C) Point and 95% CI estimates of cumulative VE to $t = 42$ months postrandomization in subgroups defined by the level of binding antibodies to scaffolded gp70-V1V2 Env, VE($t|s$) = 1 − Vrisk($t|s$)/Prisk($t|s$) for s varying over the range of binding levels in the binding antibody multiplex assay; (B) Point and 95% CI estimates of cumulative VE against HIV-1 matched to the vaccine at Env V2 site 169 and against HIV-1 mismatched to the vaccine at Env V2 site 169, VE(t,j) = 1 − Vrisk(t,j)/Prisk(t,j), for j = match and mismatch; (D) Point and 95% CI estimates of VE($t,j|x,s$) = 1−Vrisk($t,j|x,s$)/Prisk($t,j|x,s$) to $t = 39$ months against Env V2 169-matched HIV ($j = 0$) in subgroups defined by the level s of binding antibodies to scaffolded gp70-V1V2 Env and by the baseline covariate X of whether the participant has a CC at position 126 in intron 2 of the Fc-gamma receptor 2C gene locus ($x = 0$) or has (CT or CT) at this locus ($x = 1$).

blinded on a common sample set from a random sample of trial participants who completed the trial free of the study endpoint (mostly vaccine recipients and a small number of placebo recipients). With a uniform data processing and analysis plan each assay is scored by multiple statistical criteria including high specificity to detect vaccine-induced responses, a large dynamic range of vaccine-induced immune responses, and high reproducibility on within-vaccine-recipient replicate samples. Data from external trials of the study vaccine may also be used. Based on statistical analysis of the pilot data, assays are down-selected and the IR markers to be assessed as correlates are optimized and defined. For each of several immunological classes selected based on knowledge of their potential importance for protection, this analysis identifies the best-in-class IR markers based on signal-to-noise properties, vetting many factors including which readout, which sample dilutions, how to account for antigen-control readouts, how to account for baseline readouts, how to derive a marker-combination score, and which set of pathogen antigens to use and how.[62]

Pilot studies are particularly important for high-dimensional assays including whole genome transcriptomic and mass cytometry assays that are becoming increasingly important in systems vaccinology. In this context, pilot studies provide independent data that can be used to optimize analysis strategies and define marker-combination scores that reduce the dimensionality of the data while retaining most of the biological information in the original data set. Analyses that are fully data driven and analyses that account for prior biological information can both be used to group and summarize variables to define fewer variables with biological interpretations. Fully data driven approaches include dimension reduction techniques such as principal component and factor analyses and clustering approaches for reducing the number of measured variables. Such an approach has been successfully applied to peptide microarray data generated as part of the RV144 immune correlates study, which has led to the confirmation of correlates of risk.[49,62] In this case, peptides with vaccine-induced responses were first selected by comparing pre- and postvaccination samples. Reactive peptides were then clustered by their linear positioning within the HIV envelope glycoprotein (gp160), and the most representative peptide(s) within each cluster were selected as candidate variables for correlates of risk analysis (Fig. 7.2).

In contrast, other approaches group variables (e.g., genes) based on prior biological information (e.g., pathways). For example, for RNA-seq, we may use module-based approaches to reduce the dimensionality of the data set from 10,000 + genes to a few hundred modules or gene-sets.[63,64] The number of modules can then be further reduced by selecting transcriptional changes that are vaccine specific (i.e., by comparing vaccine and placebo recipients or pre- and postvaccination samples). The original variables (e.g., individual gene profiles) could be assessed as part of secondary analyses as discussed later, perhaps after down-selection of vaccine induced changes (e.g., differentially expressed genes between vaccine and placebo recipients).

Correlates of Risk and Correlates of Protection Analysis

A correlate of risk (CoR) is an IR marker S measured from vaccine or placebo recipients that is statistically associated with the rate of the study endpoint.[65] Qin et al.[65] and Plotkin and Gilbert[66] defined a correlate of protection (CoP) as an IR marker S in vaccine recipients that is a strong effect modifier of VE(t), i.e., VE($t|s$) varies over subgroups defined by levels $S = s$ of the marker. CoRs and CoPs can each be divided into two types, "fixed time" and "time-dependent" correlates. A fixed time CoR is a marker S measured at the fixed time point τ (typically postimmunizations) that is associated with

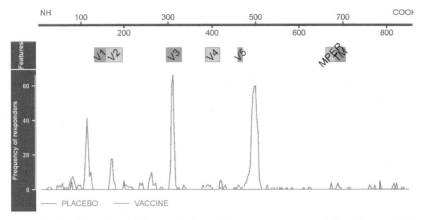

FIGURE 7.2 Illustration of down-selection of immune response variables from a high-dimensional peptide microarray assay in the RV144 immune correlates study. A set of 100 samples (20 placebo recipients, 80 vaccine recipients) pre- and postvaccination were used in a pilot study to identify immunogenic regions and select a single peptide to represent each region. Percentage of subjects with positive response after vaccination (y-axis) at position p in HXB2 alignment (x-axis) within the HIV envelope glycoprotein (gp160) broken down by vaccination status. Four hotspot regions are observed, denoted as C1, V2, V3, and C5. Peptide sequences centered at the maximum response within each major reactive region were used as candidate variables for correlates of risk analysis.

subsequent occurrence of the endpoint by time t (with $\tau < t$), while a time-dependent CoR is a marker S measured over time such that the current level of S associates with the instantaneous incidence of the endpoint at that time. Fixed time and time-dependent CoPs are defined in a parallel fashion as effect modifiers of cumulative VE or instantaneous VE, respectively. As such, validated fixed time CoPs can be used as surrogate (i.e., replacement) endpoints for the clinically significant infection study endpoint without needing to measure the study endpoint,[67] and the most practicable surrogates are measured close to entry into the study, allowing VE to be inferred with short-term follow-up trials. Therefore, development of innate response signatures within hours or days of first vaccination[68] is a promising area of correlates research. In particular, whole genome transcriptomic assays including gene expression microarrays and RNA-seq have become important tools for studying innate immune responses and identifying correlates of adaptive responses or VE as they provide a rapid and unbiased view of early expression changes after vaccination. These technologies have already been applied to identify signatures of disease progression and vaccine efficacy in the context of yellow fever,[68,69] lupus,[63] and flu[70,71] to name a few disease areas.

Importantly, a fixed time IR may be an excellent surrogate endpoint, allowing statistical prediction of VE(t)—even if it is not a mechanism of protection—which has been called a nonmechanistic CoP.[66] On the other hand, time-dependent CoPs cannot be used as surrogate endpoints, because their assessment requires longitudinal measurements throughout study follow-up. Rather, their utility is primarily to generate clues and hypotheses about the mechanistic correlates of protection, as the immune response at the time of exposure may be most relevant to a mechanism of protection (and is akin to CoP assessment in a challenge trial that attempts to approximate an exposure-conditional VE parameter).

Statistically, a CoR in vaccine recipients is identified through analysis showing that Vrisk($t|s$) significantly varies in the level of the marker s, and a CoP is identified through analysis showing that VE($t|s$) significantly varies in s. In each case it is important to estimate the whole curves Vrisk($t|s$) and VE($t|s$) over all levels s in order to fully characterize the CoR or CoP, for one or more fixed times t. Typically t is selected to be near the end of follow up, and earlier time points may also be studied to assess if and how the association changes with time.[72] We now summarize some major statistical challenges posed to estimation of Vrisk($t|s$) and VE($t|s$), focusing on the scenario where S is measured at the fixed time point $\tau < t$.

Vrisk($t|s$) is typically estimated based on measurements of S from all participants who acquire the study endpoint after τ through to time t (cases), and measurements of S from a random sample of participants who complete the follow-up period free of the study endpoint (controls). A regression model is often used such as logistic regression or Cox regression. Special versions of these methods are used that employ inverse probability weighting of participants to assure an unbiased estimate of Vrisk($t|s$), correcting for the fact that the ratio of cases to controls with S measured is greater than the ratio of all cases to all controls (e.g., Refs. 73,74). Statistical challenges for assessing CoRs include:

1. How many and which participants to select for measurement of S?
2. How to account for the signal-to-noise ratio of S?
3. How to correctly model the functional shape of Risk($t|s$) as a function of s?
4. How to assess Risk($t|s$) when S is high-dimensional such as in systems vaccinology analysis?

For issue 1, typically a random sample of two to five times as many controls per cases is used, with simulation studies conducted to understand the statistical power tradeoffs of different controls:cases ratios compared to the gold standard design that measures S in all control participants. If there are participant factors X measured in everyone that are highly correlated with S, then the sampling design can be made more statistically efficient by over-sampling subgroups that maximize the variability in S (e.g., by over-sampling subgroups with low predicted S and with high predicted S).[75] For issue 2, the fraction ρ of inter-vaccinee variability of the IR marker that is not plausibly relevant for protection has a major impact to reduce statistical power for detecting a CoR. Such protection-irrelevant variability can arise due to multiple factors including technical measurement error of the assay or variability in the number of days between the last immunization and specimen sampling for measuring S. Therefore, only validated or qualified assays documented to have adequately high ρ are warranted for inclusion in correlates studies, and, ideally, information on ρ will be used to qualify assays. (Therefore an objective of the pilot studies is to characterize ρ.) Moreover, the power calculations for detecting CoRs should explicitly consider the measurement error issue, e.g., by conducting the power calculations for a range of specified values of ρ.[56,76]

For issue 3, goodness-of-fit techniques for checking regression modeling assumptions for different forms of multivariate S may be used, which require care to ensure they properly handle the nested case-control or case-cohort sampling designs. Given that many immune CoPs for licensed vaccines used by the U.S. FDA are dichotomous indicator variables of whether an immune response readout exceeds a threshold, of particular interest is "threshold searching" methods that select the cut-point of response that creates the strongest dichotomous predictor of the study endpoint.[77] For issue 4, we recommend the use of a pilot study as described above to down select the most informative variables or variable combination by using an independent data set. However, even in this case, it is likely that a given high-dimensional assay will lead to a large number of variables that will need to be assessed as CoRs. Supervised learning model selection methods may be used that select the set of markers S and the mathematical function for combining them that best predict the study endpoint, where "best prediction" is defined based on estimated prediction accuracy for data held out of the model building, e.g., through cross-validation.[78,79] One such example is the use of a penalized regression model (e.g., logistic or Cox) where a constraint is placed on the regression coefficients to encourage the selection of a parsimonious model with fewer variables.[80,81] These supervised approaches are advantageous as they maximize objectivity in the identification of the most predictive combination IR marker. However, they typically require a large number of endpoint cases to perform well, suggesting they may be best placed for large Phase 3 trials or meta-analysis of multiple efficacy trials. Second, unsupervised learning model selection methods may be used that analyze S ignoring the endpoint data, to derive a low-dimensional summary IR marker S^* discriminating subgroups that would then be assessed as a CoR. This would be similar to what we have described above in the context of the pilot study. For example, in the presence of pre-vaccination samples—which we typically recommend for high-dimensional assays to minimize technical variation[82]— one could down-select immune markers that are vaccine induced. An alternative would be to let S^* be clusters identified through hierarchical clustering or K-means clustering, or could be the top one to three principal components based on S, possibly estimated using a method that is robust to outliers that could be caused by lab errors.[83] In practice both supervised and unsupervised learning approaches are useful and complementary.

For fixed time CoP assessment, VE($t|s$) is estimated based on the same data used for Vrisk($t|s$), plus the data from placebo recipients for estimating Prisk($t|s$), which can be done more accurately and precisely by using the "baseline immunogenicity predictor" (BIP) and/or "close-out placebo vaccination" (CPV) strategies.[84] The BIP strategy measures participant characteristics at baseline and uses them to predict the values S of placebo recipients that they would have had if, contrary to fact, they had been assigned to receive the vaccine. The CPV strategy measures these values of S directly after giving placebo recipients the vaccine once they complete the trial free of the endpoint. Several statistical methods have been developed for estimating VE($t|s$) based on the BIP and/or CPV strategies, including.[46,72,84,85] Gilbert et al.[86] illustrates an application of the BIP approach for assessing a fixed time CoP in a varicella zoster vaccine efficacy trial.

Statistical challenges for assessing CoPs include all of those for assessing CoRs plus additional challenges including:

1. How to develop baseline immunogenicity predictors (BIPs) of the IR marker S to vaccination?
2. How many and which participants to select for measuring BIPs and for undergoing CPV?
3. How to do sensitivity analysis accounting for the fact that not all assumptions needed for estimating VE($t|s$) can be fully verified?

Issue 1 may be studied by statistical association analyses in the efficacy trial or in other vaccine studies, e.g., studying the following types of baseline characteristics as BIPs: demographics, the IR marker S measured at baseline,[72,86] innate immunity gene expression profiles,[68] cell population frequencies measure at multiple baseline/pre-vaccination time points[87] immune responses to the vector carrying the pathogen insert (if a vector-based vaccine), or immune responses to a different vaccine that is licensed and is unlikely to affect the risk of the study endpoint after accounting for the marker S and is unlikely to affect the efficacy of the vaccine under study.[84,88] For issue 2, a first decision is whether to use CPV at all. To our knowledge it has never been used; however, it is appealing if applied adaptively after the trial establishes beneficial vaccine efficacy, for in that case it becomes important to study immune correlates of protection and benefit is provided to placebo recipients by offering them the vaccine in a timely manner.[56] If feasible, CPV is also recommended because it provides a way to test the modeling assumptions made for estimating Prisk($t|S$). If CPV is used, a next decision is how many and which placebo recipients to offer CPV, combined with the decision of how many and which vaccine and placebo recipients to measure the BIPs. A decision analysis may be used that optimizes the statistical efficiency for estimating VE(t|s) conditional on a fixed amount of resources available for measuring S and BIPs.[85] For issue 3, a principled approach would report "ignorance intervals" and "estimated uncertainty intervals" for the curve VE(t|s), where ignorance intervals are the range of point estimates obtained under the range of plausible violations of the not fully verifiable assumption(s) and estimated uncertainty intervals are the union of confidence intervals under this range of possible violations.[61,89] Estimated uncertainty intervals provide a more accurate envelope indicating where the true curve VE(t|s) may lie compared to confidence intervals that optimistically assume the unverifiable assumption(s) is true. Fig. 7.1B illustrates estimation of VE(t|s) for the RV144 HIV vaccine efficacy trial.

For X a baseline covariate, it is relatively straightforward to estimate VE(t|x) over subgroups x to study effect modification. If X is measured in everyone then standard survival analysis methods may be used, and if X is measured in a random sample, then similar methods used for CoR assessment may be used. If X is expensive such as host genetics or other metagenomics data, and the rate of the study endpoint is rare (e.g., less than 15% of trial participants experience the endpoint), then the case-only method is highly advantageous for estimating VE(t|x), because it only requires measuring X in disease cases, and it is statistically efficient compared to designs that also include data on X from controls.[90,91]

STATISTICAL ISSUES IN ASSESSING IMMUNE CORRELATES OF PROTECTION VIA ESTIMATION OF VE(t,j) OR VE(t,j | x)

Genotypic Sieve Analysis

Genotypic sieve analysis assesses if and how VE to prevent the study endpoint depends on nucleotide or amino acid features of the pathogen exposing trial participants.[92] Two major types of sieve analysis include: (1) (Local) Assessment of if and how VE differs against vaccine-matched versus vaccine-mismatched genotypes of the pathogen, with genotype defined by a single amino acid position, a known or predicted epitope, or some other set of amino acids and (2) (Global) Assessment of if and how VE differs against pathogens with different amino acid distances (based on a protein or protein region) to the sequence(s) in the vaccine. Analysis of differential VE by genotype may be conducted using survival analysis regression methods (e.g., Ref. 93) and on supervised learning model selection methods for predicting vaccination status from genotypic pathogen features (e.g., Refs. 79,94). Edlefsen et al.[94] summarize a variety of statistical approaches to the two types of sieve analysis. Statistical challenges posed to genotypic sieve analysis include:

1. Interpretability of a sieve analysis requires that the pathogen genotype feature be known at the time of pathogen acquisition/infection. For genetically diverse pathogens that rapidly evolve postacquisition, how can the

analysis address the fact that sequences from some participants are measured after acquisition?

2. How to account for the fact that multiple pathogens may establish infection within some individuals?
3. The most informative sieve analyses focus on immunologically relevant amino acid sites or sets of sites of the pathogen for the vaccine under study. How to account for information on vaccine-induced immune responses and on the structure of the pathogen?

Issue 1 is moot for pathogens with minimal evolution in the first several months after acquisition (e.g., malaria, dengue), but is important for fast-evolving pathogens such as HIV-1. Where it is relevant, one approach incorporates models predictive of infecting sequences into the method for estimating $VE(t,j)$,[93] e.g., built with phylogenetic methods.[95] Issue 2 may be addressed by focusing the sieve analysis on amino acid sites that satisfy a certain immuno-virological criterion, e.g., being in an epitope target of measured vaccine immune responses[49] or being known or predicted to be on the outer surface of the pathogen and potentially accessible to antibodies. Fig. 7.1C illustrates estimation of $VE(t,j)$ for the RV144 HIV-1 vaccine efficacy trial, for j = match or mismatch to the vaccine at amino acid position 169 in the V2 region of HIV-1 Envelope.

For X a baseline covariate, if X is measured in everyone then $VE(t,j|x)$ may be studied using the same methods as described above, and if X is measured in a random sample, then $VE(t,j|x)$ may be studied using similar methods augmented with inverse probability weighting (as for CoR analyses). Li et al.[96] illustrate application of the case-only method[97] to the RV144 trial; they estimated $VE(t,j|x)$ with j = match or mismatch to the vaccine at amino acid position 169 in the V2 region of HIV-1 Envelope and X data from SNP analysis of Fc gamma receptor genes.

Phenotypic Sieve Analysis

Phenotypic sieve analysis compares between the infected vaccine and infected placebo case groups the sensitivity of the breakthrough infecting pathogens as determined by an immunological assay such as neutralization.[98] For example, for the Vax004 HIV-1 vaccine efficacy trial, HIV-1 Envelope gp120 pseudo-viruses were made from breakthrough infected vaccine and placebo recipients, and the sensitivity to neutralization of each pseudo-virus was measured based on TZM-bl assay measurements from preinfection blood samples of vaccine recipients.[99] Reduced neutralization sensitivity of breakthrough viruses in vaccine recipients compared to placebo recipients would suggest that the vaccine selectively blocked infections with neutralization sensitive variants. Conducting the phenotypic sieve analysis for a set of assays measuring different potential protective functions (e.g., neutralization and assays measuring Fc effector functions) provides an empirical basis for discriminating which types of responses are more or less associated with vaccine efficacy. While this approach is conceptually promising, it appears to have seldom been used; however with improvements in technology for making antigen reagent panels it merits more attention in future vaccine efficacy trials.

ASSESSING IMMUNE CORRELATES OF PROTECTION VIA ESTIMATION OF VE($t,j\,|\,s$)

Sieve analysis is a tightly integrated component of immune correlates assessment, as the "other side of the same coin." On the heads side, sieve analysis can be used to validate whether an immunological measurement is a CoP. To illustrate, suppose the vaccine partially protects (VE(t) > 0%) and the correlates analysis points to neutralizing antibody titers to a specific protein of the pathogen as a potential CoP. If these titers are indeed a good CoP, then we would expect to observe greater sequence distances to the vaccine-insert sequence (in the specific region) in infected vaccine recipients compared to infected placebo recipients. Sieve analysis provides a test of this hypothesis. On the tails side of the coin, if the vaccine partially protects (VE(t) > 0%) and the sieve analysis detects sequence differences vaccine versus placebo in a specific pathogen region, then it follows that the vaccine must have placed immune pressure on the pathogen (because the trial is randomized and double-blinded). This finding would generate the hypothesis that IR markers measuring immune responses to the specific pathogen region are CoPs, thereby guiding the definition of antigen-specific IR markers to assess as CoPs. Therefore, sieve analysis can both help corroborate immune CoPs and guide the definition of immune variables to evaluate as CoPs. These concepts may be implemented empirically by estimating VE($t,j\,|\,s$) for specific paired choices of the IR marker s and the pathogen feature j, e.g., in dengue vaccine efficacy trials it is of interest to assess serotype-specific neutralization titers as CoPs for serotype-specific dengue disease.[18,60] For a second example, the RV144 trial assessed VE($t = 42$ months,$j\,|\,s$) for IgG binding antibody levels to gp70 scaffolded HIV-1 Envelope V1V2 proteins paired with whether the HIV-1 had a vaccine-matched or mismatched residue at site 169 in V2.[96,100] Moreover, the analysis may be done in baseline subgroups X, and Fig. 7.1D illustrates estimation of VE($t,j\,|\,x,s$) in RV144 using the same data as in Fig. 7.1A and B with X defined from Fc-gamma receptor genetics.[96]

In general, it is of great scientific interest to understand VE($t,j\,|\,s$) over the whole range of values of t, j, and s, and a major challenge is having enough data for precise estimation. Generally a very large Phase 3 trial or meta-analysis of multiple efficacy trials is required for direct empirical assessment of this objective. Moreover, because the immune responses that are valid surrogate endpoints may differ for different vaccine regimens, study populations, and/or pathogen populations,[67] an objective of meta-analyses is to assess the consistency of VE($t,j|s$) across settings.

ACKNOWLEDGMENTS

The authors thank Michal Juraska and Ying Huang for the data analysis producing Fig. 7.1, and Margo Rogers for help with references. This research was supported by the National Institute of Allergy and Infectious Diseases of the National Institutes of Health under Award Numbers R37AI054165 and UM1AI068635.

REFERENCES

1. Halloran ME, Longini IM, Struchiner CJ. Design and interpretation of vaccine field studies. *Epidemiol Rev* 1999;**21**(1):73–88.
2. Halloran ME, Longini IM, Struchiner CJ. In: Gail M, Krickelberg K, Samet J, Tsiatis A, Wong W, editors. *Design and analysis of vaccine studies*. New York: Springer; 2010.
3. Hudgens MG, Gilbert PB, Self SG. Endpoints in vaccine trials. *Stat Methods Med Res* 2004;**13**(2):89–114.
4. Hussey MA, Hughes JP. Design and analysis of stepped wedge cluster randomized trials. *Contemp Clin Trials* 2007;**28**(2):182–91.
5. Moulton LH, Golub JE, Durovni B, Cavalcante SC, Pacheco AG, Saraceni V, et al. Statistical design of THRio: a phased implementation clinic-randomized study of a tuberculosis preventive therapy intervention. *Clin Trials* 2007;**4**(2):190–9.
6. Moulton LH, O'Brien KL, Reid R, Weatherholtz R, Santosham M, Siber GR. Evaluation of the indirect effects of a pneumococcal vaccine in a community-randomized study. *J Biopharm Stat* 2006;**16**(4):453–62.
7. The Gambia Hepatitis Intervention Study. The Gambia Hepatitis Study Group. *Cancer Res* 1987;**47**(21):5782–7.
8. Brown CA, Lilford RJ. The stepped wedge trial design: a systematic review. *BMC Med Res Methodol* 2006;**6**:54. PMCID: 1636652.
9. Stephens AJ, Tchetgen Tchetgen EJ, De Gruttola V. Augmented generalized estimating equations for improving efficiency and validity of estimation in cluster randomized trials by leveraging cluster-level and individual-level covariates. *Stat Med* 2012;**31**(10):915–30. PMCID: 3495191.
10. Scott JM, deCamp A, Juraska M, Fay MP, Gilbert PB. Finite-sample corrected generalized estimating equation of population average treatment effects in stepped wedge cluster randomized trials. *Stat Methods Med Res* 2014.
11. Hayes RJ, Moulton LH. In: Chow S-C, Peace KE, Liu J-P, Jones B, Turnbull BW, editors. *Cluster randomised trials*. New York: Chapman & Hall/CRC Press; 2009.
12. Schaper C, Fleming TR, Self SG, Rida WN. Statistical issues in the design of HIV vaccine trials. *Annu Rev Public Health* 1995;**16**:1–22.
13. Clemens J, Brenner R, Rao M, Tafari N, Lowe C. Evaluating new vaccines for developing countries. Efficacy or effectiveness? *JAMA* 1996;**275**(5):390–7.
14. Orenstein WA, Bernier RH, Dondero TJ, Hinman AR, Marks JS, Bart KJ, et al. Field evaluation of vaccine efficacy. *Bull World Health Organ* 1985;**63**(6):1055–68. PMCID: 2536484.

15. Rida WN, Lawrence DN. Some statistical issues in HIV vaccine trials. *Stat Med* 1994;**13** (19−20):2155−77.

16. Foppa IM, Haber M, Ferdinands JM, Shay DK. The case test-negative design for studies of the effectiveness of influenza vaccine. *Vaccine* 2013;**31**(30):3104−9.

17. Rida W, Fast P, Hoff R, Fleming T. Intermediate-size trials for the evaluation of HIV vaccine candidates: a workshop summary. *J Acquir Immune Defic Syndr Hum Retrovirol* 1997;**16**(3):195−203.

18. Sabchareon A, Wallace D, Sirivichayakul C, Limkittikul K, Chanthavanich P, Suvannadabba S, et al. Protective efficacy of the recombinant, live-attenuated, CYD tetravalent dengue vaccine in Thai schoolchildren: a randomised, controlled phase 2b trial. *Lancet* 2012;**380**(9853):1559−67.

19. Excler JL, Rida W, Priddy F, Fast P, Koff W. A strategy for accelerating the development of preventive AIDS vaccines. *AIDS* 2007;**21**(17):2259−63.

20. Gilbert PB. Some design issues in phase 2B vs phase 3 prevention trials for testing efficacy of products or concepts. *Stat Med* 2010;**29**(10):1061−71. PMCID: 2929839.

21. Clements-Mann ML. Lessons for AIDS vaccine development from non-AIDS vaccines. *AIDS Res Hum Retroviruses* 1998;**14**(Suppl. 3):S197−203.

22. Hawn TR, Day TA, Scriba TJ, Hatherill M, Hanekom WA, Evans TG, et al. Tuberculosis vaccines and prevention of infection. *Microbiol Mol Biol Rev* 2014;**78**(4):650−71. PMCID: 4248657.

23. Roestenberg M, McCall M, Hopman J, Wiersma J, Luty AJ, van Gemert GJ, et al. Protection against a malaria challenge by sporozoite inoculation. *N Engl J Med* 2009;**361** (5):468−77.

24. Sauerwein RW, Roestenberg M, Moorthy VS. Experimental human challenge infections can accelerate clinical malaria vaccine development. *Nat Rev Immunol* 2011;**11**(1):57−64.

25. Talley AK, Healy SA, Finney OC, Murphy SC, Kublin J, Salas CJ, et al. Safety and comparability of controlled human *Plasmodium falciparum* infection by mosquito bite in malaria-naive subjects at a new facility for sporozoite challenge. *PLoS One* 2014;**9**(11): e109654. PMCID: 4236046.

26. Datta S, Halloran ME, Longini Jr. IM. Efficiency of estimating vaccine efficacy for susceptibility and infectiousness: randomization by individual versus household. *Biometrics* 1999;**55**(3):792−8.

27. Longini IM, Datta S, Halloran ME. Measuring vaccine efficacy for both susceptibility to infection and reduction in infectiousness for prophylactic HIV-1 vaccines. *J Acquir Immune Defic Syndr Hum Retrovirol* 1996;**13**(5):440−7.

28. Datta S, Halloran ME, Longini Jr. IM. Augmented HIV vaccine trial design for estimating reduction in infectiousness and protective efficacy. *Stat Med* 1998;**17**(2):185−200.

29. Longini Jr. IM, Hudgens MG, Halloran ME, Sagatelian K. A Markov model for measuring vaccine efficacy for both susceptibility to infection and reduction in infectiousness for prophylactic HIV vaccines. *Stat Med* 1999;**18**(1):53−68.

30. Longini IM, Hudgens MG, Halloran ME. Estimation of vaccine efficacy for both susceptibility to infection and reduction in infectiousness for prophylactic HIV vaccines with partner augmentation. In: Kaplan E, Brookmeyer R, editors. *The quantitative evaluation of HIV prevention programs.* New Haven, CT: Yale University Press; 2002. p. 241−59.

31. Greenwood M, Yule GU. The statistics of anti-typhoid and anti-cholera inoculations, and the interpretation of such statistics in general. In: *Proc R Soc Med.* 1915;**8**(Sect Epidemiol State Med):113−194. PMCID: 2004181.

32. Rhodes PH, Halloran ME, Longini IM. Counting process models for infectious disease data: distinguishing exposure to infection from susceptibility. *J R Statist Soc B* 1996;**58** (4):751−62.

33. Golm GT, Halloran ME, Longini IM. Validation sets for exposure to infection in HIV vaccine trials.... In: *Proceedings of the epidemiology section of the American Statistical Association; Dallas, TX*; 1998.

34. Halloran ME, Longini Jr. IM. Using validation sets for outcomes and exposure to infection in vaccine field studies. *Am J Epidemiol* 2001;**154**(5):391−8.

35. Yang Y, Halloran ME, Longini Jr. IM. A Bayesian model for evaluating influenza antiviral efficacy in household studies with asymptomatic infections. *Biostatistics* 2009;**10** (2):390−403. PMCID: 2733175.

36. Yang Y, Longini IM, Halloran ME. Design and evaluation of prophylactic interventions using infectious disease incidence data from close contact groups. *J R Stat Soc Ser C Appl Stat* 2006;**55**:317−30.

37. Dimitrov D, Donnell D, Brown ER. High incidence is not high exposure: what proportion of prevention trial participants are exposed to HIV? *PLoS One* 2015;**10**(1):e0115528. PMCID: 4287619.

38. Trollfors B, Taranger J, Lagergard T, Lind L, Sundh V, Zackrisson G, et al. A placebo-controlled trial of a pertussis-toxoid vaccine. *N Engl J Med* 1995;**333**(16):1045−50.

39. Vrijens B, Urquhart J. Patient adherence to prescribed antimicrobial drug dosing regimens. *J Antimicrob Chemother* 2005;**55**(5):616−27.

40. Smith PG, Rodrigues LC, Fine PE. Assessment of the protective efficacy of vaccines against common diseases using case-control and cohort studies. *Int J Epidemiol* 1984;**13**(1):87−93.

41. Zhang M, Tsiatis AA, Davidian M. Improving efficiency of inferences in randomized clinical trials using auxiliary covariates. *Biometrics* 2008;**64**(3):707−15. PMCID: 2574960.

42. Moore KL, van der Laan MJ. Increasing power in randomized trials with right censored outcomes through covariate adjustment. *J Biopharm Stat* 2009;**19**(6):1099−131. PMCID: 2895464.

43. van der Laan MJ, Rose S. *Targeted learning: causal inference for observational and experimental data*. New York: Springer; 2011.

44. Hernan MA. The hazards of hazard ratios. *Epidemiology* 2010;**21**(1):13−15. PMCID: 3653612.

45. Stitelman OM, Wester CW, De Gruttola V, van der Laan MJ. Targeted maximum likelihood estimation of effect modification parameters in survival analysis. *Int J Biostat* 2011;**7** (1):19. PMCID: 3083138.

46. Gilbert PB, Hudgens MG. Evaluating candidate principal surrogate endpoints. *Biometrics* 2008;**64**(4):1146−54. PMCID: 2726718.

47. Briney BS, Willis JR, McKinney BA, Crowe Jr. JE. High-throughput antibody sequencing reveals genetic evidence of global regulation of the naive and memory repertoires that extends across individuals. *Genes Immun* 2012;**13**(6):469−73.

48. Brown EP, Licht AF, Dugast AS, Choi I, Bailey-Kellogg C, Alter G, et al. High-throughput, multiplexed IgG subclassing of antigen-specific antibodies from clinical samples. *J Immunol Methods* 2012;**386**(1−2):117−23. PMCID: 3475184.

49. Gottardo R, Bailer RT, Korber BT, Gnanakaran S, Phillips J, Shen X, et al. Plasma IgG to linear epitopes in the V2 and V3 regions of HIV-1 gp120 correlate with a reduced risk of infection in the RV144 vaccine efficacy trial. *PLoS One* 2013;**8**(9):e75665. PMCID: 3784573.

50. Mascola JR, D'Souza P, Gilbert P, Hahn BH, Haigwood NL, Morris L, et al. Recommendations for the design and use of standard virus panels to assess neutralizing antibody responses elicited by candidate human immunodeficiency virus type 1 vaccines. *J Virol* 2005;**79**(16):10103−7. PMCID: 1182642.

51. Seaman MS, Janes H, Hawkins N, Grandpre LE, Devoy C, Giri A, et al. Tiered categorization of a diverse panel of HIV-1 Env pseudoviruses for assessment of neutralizing antibodies. *J Virol* 2010;**84**(3):1439−52. PMCID: 2812321.

52. deCamp A, Hraber P, Bailer RT, Seaman MS, Ochsenbauer C, Kappes J, et al. Global panel of HIV-1 Env reference strains for standardized assessments of vaccine-elicited neutralizing antibodies. *J Virol* 2014;**88**(5):2489−507. PMCID: 3958090.

53. Hudgens MG, Halloran ME. Toward causal inference with interference. *J Am Stat Assoc* 2008;**103**(482):832−42. PMCID: 2600548.

54. Tchetgen EJ, VanderWeele TJ. On causal inference in the presence of interference. *Stat Methods Med Res* 2012;**21**(1):55−75. PMCID: 4216807.

55. Ellenberg SS, Fleming TR, DeMets DL. *Data monitoring committees in clinical trials: a practical perspective.* New York: John Wiley & Sons; 2002.

56. Gilbert PB, Grove D, Gabriel E, Huang Y, Gray G, Hammer SM, et al. A sequential phase 2b trial design for evaluating vaccine efficacy and immune correlates for multiple HIV vaccine regimens. *Stat Commun Infect Dis* 2011;**3**(1). PMCID: Pmc3502884.

57. Juraska M, Grove D. seqDesign: simulation and group sequential monitoring of randomized multi-arm two-stage Phase IIb/III treatment efficacy trials with time-to-event endpoints. R package, Comprehensive R Archive Network; 2014.

58. Horne AD, Lachenbruch PA, Goldenthal KL. Intent-to-treat analysis and preventive vaccine efficacy. *Vaccine* 2000;**19**(2−3):319−26.

59. Gilbert PB, Berger JO, Stablein D, Becker S, Essex M, Hammer SM, et al. Statistical interpretation of the RV144 HIV vaccine efficacy trial in Thailand: a case study for statistical issues in efficacy trials. *J Infect Dis* 2011;**203**(7):969−75. PMCID: 3068028.

60. Capeding MR, Tran NH, Hadinegoro SR, Ismail HI, Chotpitayasunondh T, Chua MN, et al. Clinical efficacy and safety of a novel tetravalent dengue vaccine in healthy children in Asia: a phase 3, randomised, observer-masked, placebo-controlled trial. *Lancet* 2014;**384**(9951):1358−65.

61. Gilbert PB, Shepherd BE, Hudgens MG. Sensitivity analysis of per-protocol time-to-event treatment efficacy in randomized clinical trials. *J Am Stat Assoc* 2013;**108**(503). PMCID: 3811958.

62. Haynes BF, Gilbert PB, McElrath MJ, Zolla-Pazner S, Tomaras GD, Alam SM, et al. Immune-correlates analysis of an HIV-1 vaccine efficacy trial. *N Engl J Med* 2012;**366**(14):1275−86. PMCID: 3371689.

63. Chaussabel D, Quinn C, Shen J, Patel P, Glaser C, Baldwin N, et al. A modular analysis framework for blood genomics studies: application to systemic lupus erythematosus. *Immunity* 2008;**29**(1):150−64. PMCID: 2727981.

64. Li S, Rouphael N, Duraisingham S, Romero-Steiner S, Presnell S, Davis C, et al. Molecular signatures of antibody responses derived from a systems biology study of five human vaccines. *Nat Immunol* 2014;**15**(2):195−204. PMCID: 3946932.

65. Qin L, Gilbert PB, Corey L, McElrath MJ, Self SG. A framework for assessing immunological correlates of protection in vaccine trials. *J Infect Dis* 2007;**196**(9):1304−12.

66. Plotkin SA, Gilbert PB. Nomenclature for immune correlates of protection after vaccination. *Clin Infect Dis* 2012;**54**(11):1615−17. PMCID: 3348952.

67. Fleming TR, Powers JH. Biomarkers and surrogate endpoints in clinical trials. *Stat Med* 2012;**31**(25):2973−84. PMCID: 3551627.

68. Querec TD, Akondy RS, Lee EK, Cao W, Nakaya HI, Teuwen D, et al. Systems biology approach predicts immunogenicity of the yellow fever vaccine in humans. *Nat Immunol* 2009;**10**(1):116−25. PMCID: 4049462.

69. Gaucher D, Therrien R, Kettaf N, Angermann BR, Boucher G, Filali-Mouhim A, et al. Yellow fever vaccine induces integrated multilineage and polyfunctional immune responses. *J Exp Med* 2008;**205**(13):3119−31. PMCID: 2605227.

70. Nakaya HI, Wrammert J, Lee EK, Racioppi L, Marie-Kunze S, Haining WN, et al. Systems biology of vaccination for seasonal influenza in humans. *Nat Immunol* 2011;**12**(8):786−95. PMCID: 3140559.

71. Furman D, Jojic V, Kidd B, Shen-Orr S, Price J, Jarrell J, et al. Apoptosis and other immune biomarkers predict influenza vaccine responsiveness. *Mol Syst Biol* 2013;**9**:659. PMCID: 3658270.

72. Gabriel EE, Gilbert PB. Evaluating principal surrogate endpoints with time-to-event data accounting for time-varying treatment efficacy. *Biostatistics* 2014;**15**(2):251−65. PMCID: 3944974.

73. Prentice RL. A case-cohort design for epidemiologic cohort studies and disease prevention trials. *Biometrika* 1986;**73**(1):1−11.

74. Borgan O, Langholz B, Samuelsen SO, Goldstein L, Pogoda J. Exposure stratified case-cohort designs. *Lifetime Data Anal* 2000;**6**(1):39−58.

75. Breslow NE, Lumley T, Ballantyne CM, Chambless LE, Kulich M. Using the whole cohort in the analysis of case-cohort data. *Am J Epidemiol* 2009;**169**(11):1398−405. PMCID: 2768499.

76. Gilbert PB, Janes HE, Huang Y. Power/sample size calculations for assessing correlates of risk in clinical efficacy trials. *Statistics in Medicine* 2016. PMID: 27037797. *Epublished ahead of print. DOI: 10.1002/sim. 6952.*

77. Fong Y, Di C, Permar S. Change point testing in logistic regression models with interaction term. *Stat Med* 2015.

78. James G, Witten D, Hastie T, Ribshirani R. In: Casella G, Fienberg S, Olkin I, editors. *An introduction to statistical learning.* New York: Springer; 2013.

79. van der Laan MJ, Polley EC, Hubbard AE. Super learner. *Stat Appl Genet Mol Biol* 2007;**6**:Article25.

80. Gui J, Li H. Penalized Cox regression analysis in the high-dimensional and low-sample size settings, with applications to microarray gene expression data. *Bioinformatics* 2005;**21**(13):3001−8.

81. Tibshirani R. Regression shrinkage and selection via the Lasso. *J R Statist Soc B* 1996;**58**(1):267−88.

82. Imholte GC, Sauteraud R, Korber B, Bailer RT, Turk ET, Shen X, et al. A computational framework for the analysis of peptide microarray antibody binding data with application to HIV vaccine profiling. *J Immunol Methods* 2013;**395**(1−2):1−13. PMCID: 3999921.

83. Candes EJ, Li XD, Ma Y, Wright J. Robust principal component analysis? *J ACM* 2011;**58**(3).

84. Follmann D. Augmented designs to assess immune response in vaccine trials. *Biometrics* 2006;**62**(4):1161−9. PMCID: 2536776.

85. Huang Y, Gilbert PB, Wolfson J. Design and estimation for evaluating principal surrogate markers in vaccine trials. *Biometrics* 2013;**69**(2):301−9. PMCID: 3713795.

86. Gilbert PB, Gabriel EE, Miao X, Li X, Su SC, Parrino J, et al. Fold rise in antibody titers by measured by glycoprotein-based enzyme-linked immunosorbent assay is an excellent correlate of protection for a herpes zoster vaccine, demonstrated via the vaccine efficacy curve. *J Infect Dis* 2014;**210**(10):1573−81. PMCID: 4215071.

87. Tsang JS, Schwartzberg PL, Kotliarov Y, Biancotto A, Xie Z, Germain RN, et al. Baylor HIPC Center; CHI Consortium. Global analyses of human immune variation reveal baseline predictors of postvaccination responses. *Cell* 2014 Apr 10;**157**(2):499−513.

88. Czeschinski PA, Binding N, Witting U. Hepatitis A and hepatitis B vaccinations: immunogenicity of combined vaccine and of simultaneously or separately applied single vaccines. *Vaccine* 2000;**18**(11−12):1074−80.

89. Vansteelandt S, Goetghebeur E, Kenward MG, Molenberghs G. Ignorance and uncertainty regions as inferential tools in a sensitivity analysis. *Stat Sinica* 2006;**16**:953−79.

90. Vittinghoff E, Bauer DC. Case-only analysis of treatment-covariate interactions in clinical trials. *Biometrics* 2006;**62**(3):769−76.

91. Dai JY, Logsdon BA, Huang Y, Hsu L, Reiner AP, Prentice RL, et al. Simultaneously testing for marginal genetic association and gene-environment interaction. *Am J Epidemiol* 2012;**176**(2):164−73. PMCID: 3499112.

92. Gilbert PB, Self SG, Ashby MA. Statistical methods for assessing differential vaccine protection against human immunodeficiency virus types. *Biometrics* 1998;**54**(3):799−814.

93. Gilbert PB, Sun Y. Inferences on relative failure rates in stratified mark-specific proportional hazards models with missing marks, with application to HIV vaccine efficacy trials. *J R Stat Soc Ser C Appl Stat* 2015;**64**(1):49−73. PMCID: 4310507.

94. Edlefsen PT, Rolland M, Hertz T, Tovanabutra S, Gartland AJ, deCamp AC, et al. Comprehensive sieve analysis of breakthrough HIV-1 sequences in the RV144 vaccine efficacy trial. *PLoS Comput Biol* 2015;**11**(2):e1003973. PMCID: 4315437.

95. Drummond AJ, Rambaut A. BEAST: Bayesian evolutionary analysis by sampling trees. *BMC Evol Biol* 2007;**7**:214. PMCID: 2247476.

96. Li SS, Gilbert PB, Tomaras GD, Kijak G, Ferrari G, Thomas R, et al. FCGR2C polymorphisms associate with HIV-1 vaccine protection in RV144 trial. *J Clin Invest* 2014;**124**(9):3879−90. PMCID: 4151214.

97. Dai JY, Li SS, Gilbert PB. Case-only method for cause-specific hazards models with application to assessing differential vaccine efficacy by viral and host genetics. *Biostatistics* 2014;**15**(1):196−203. PMCID: 3862206.

98. Montefiori DC. Importance of neutralization sieve analyses when seeking correlates of HIV-1 vaccine efficacy. *Hum Vaccin Immunother* 2014;**10**(8):2507−11.

99. Gilbert P, Wang M, Wrin T, Petropoulos C, Gurwith M, Sinangil F, et al. Magnitude and breadth of a nonprotective neutralizing antibody response in an efficacy trial of a candidate HIV-1 gp120 vaccine. *J Infect Dis* 2010;**202**(4):595−605. PMCID: 2946208.

100. Rolland M, Edlefsen PT, Larsen BB, Tovanabutra S, Sanders-Buell E, Hertz T, et al. Increased HIV-1 vaccine efficacy against viruses with genetic signatures in Env V2. *Nature* 2012;**490**(7420):417−20. PMCID: 3551291.

Chapter 8

Vaccine Development in Special Populations

K.M. Edwards and C.B. Creech
Vanderbilt University, Nashville, TN, United States

INFANTS

The practice of early childhood immunization is not restricted to the modern era of vaccinology. Infants and young children were routinely vaccinated against variola in the 17th and 18th centuries. It is thought that Lady Mary Montagu brought the practice of variolation to England when Charles Maitland immunized her 2-year-old daughter. Due to the success of variolation in preventing smallpox morbidity and mortality, the practice became widespread and was popularized by Edward Jenner. While not without adverse consequence (as many as 2–3% of variolated infants died), the practice led to the prevention of untold numbers of smallpox cases in infants and young children.

In the last century, the oldest scientific paper to report on the vaccination of infants was published in 1911 in the *Journal of Experimental Medicine*.[1] Lucas et al. vaccinated 95 infants with an overnight culture of *Bacillus dysenteriae*, along with antiserum, to determine whether vaccination would have an impact on infant morbidity or mortality from dysentery. In general, the approach was well-tolerated and provided some protection against dysentery, which had been responsible for numerous outbreaks and infant deaths at the time. In 1921, the first human administration of Bacille Calmette Guerin (BCG) for the prevention of tuberculosis was reported.[2] Following a woman's postpartum death from tuberculosis, her healthy infant boy was given an oral dose of BCG. The child experienced no adverse events and avoided acquiring tuberculosis. In 1924, 600 infants were vaccinated with oral BCG and by 1928 more than 100,000 infants had been safely vaccinated.[3] By 1950, safer and more effective vaccines for smallpox, diphtheria, tuberculosis, and pertussis had become widely available. Over the next 30 years, as

Human Vaccines: Emerging Technologies in Design and Development.
DOI: http://dx.doi.org/10.1016/B978-0-12-802302-0.00007-8

molecular biotechnologies and product manufacturing processes became more advanced, vaccines were developed for the most significant pediatric public health threats including measles, mumps, rubella, and polio. The success of these vaccines has been unparalleled in the history of public health, as they have resulted in a massive reduction in overall morbidity and mortality (Table 8.1).

Despite the remarkable successes in vaccine development for infants, immunizations for many neonatal and childhood pathogens are still unavailable; including, but not limited to Group B streptococcus, respiratory syncytial virus (RSV) and *Staphylococcus aureus*. The challenges of developing vaccines against these pathogens for infants are many (Fig. 8.1). They include a lack of coordination between the innate and adaptive immune responses, immune interference by maternal antibodies, and immature T and B cell responses.

Impaired Coordination Between the Innate and Adaptive Immune Responses

Among immunologically naïve infants, the innate immune system is the primary mechanism of defense against new infections. Pattern recognition receptors (i.e., Toll-like receptors (TLRs)) play a prominent role in the

TABLE 8.1 Annual Morbidity Due to Common Vaccine-Preventable Diseases Recommended for Universal Use in US Children Before 1990

Disease	20th Century Morbidity[a]	1998 Morbidity[b]	Percent Decrease
Smallpox	48,164	0	100
Diphtheria	175,885	1	99.99
Pertussis	147,271	6279	95.7
Tetanus	1314	34	97.4
Poliomyelitis (paralytic)	16,316	0	100
Measles	503,282	89	99.99
Mumps	152,209	606	99.6
Rubella	47,745	345	99.3
Haemophilus influenzae type B	20,000	54	99.7

[a]Average annual numbers of cases in the several years before universal vaccine use was recommended: smallpox (1900–04); diphtheria (1920–22); pertussis (1922–25); tetanus (1922–26); poliomyelitis (paralytic) (1951–54); measles (1958–62); mumps (1968); rubella (1966–68); H. Influenzae type B (1985).
[b]Number of cases reported for each disease in 1998.
Source: Adapted from Morb Mortal Wkly Rep 1999;48(12):243–48.

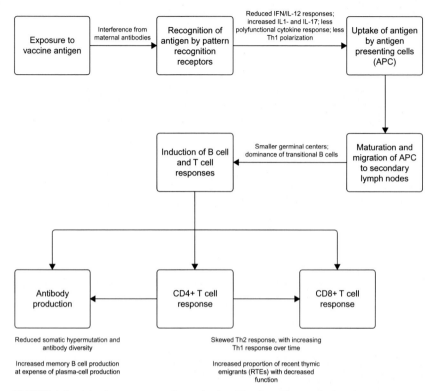

FIGURE 8.1 Adaptive response to immunization. The flow diagram depicts the general steps toward developing an adaptive immune response to a vaccine. Challenges specific to infant populations are indicated between the steps. *IFN*, interferon; *IL*, interleukin.

surveillance of an array of pathogens, including gram-negative enteric bacteria, Group B streptococcus, and respiratory viruses. Kollmann et al. demonstrated that monocytes from the peripheral blood of infants produce less interferon than monocytes from older children or adults. These infant monocytes are more adept at inducing specific T helper cell (T_h17) responses via secretion of the cytokines interleukins 6 and 23 (IL-6, IL-23).[4] In an elegant study by Shey et al., whole blood and peripheral blood mononuclear cells from newborns, 10-, and 36-week old infants were incubated with BCG or TLR ligands. Compared to older infants, BCG-induced expression of monocyte-derived, pro-inflammatory cytokines (i.e., tumor necrosis factor (TNF), IL-6, IL-12p40) was diminished in newborns. Similarly CD40 expression increased with age, as older infants had more mature signaling capacity—an effect of NF-kB on TLR1.[5] In a similar study, Lisciandro et al. evaluated innate immune responses in infants born in a resource-limited setting. The goal of the study was to determine whether early environmental exposures (e.g., parasitic infections) alter the balance of T_h1 and T_h2

responses in infants. Infant whole blood was exposed to a panel of TLR and nucleotide-binding oligomerization domain (NOD-like) receptor agonists, as well as an aluminum salt adjuvant. The adjuvant induced IL-1β and IL-8 responses that decreased with age, while inflammatory responses to TLR2 and TLR3 ligands increased (higher expression of IL-6, IL-1 β, interferon (IFN-γ)). Perhaps most importantly, the anti-inflammatory cytokine, IL-10, was preserved in this infant population. These data suggest that age-dependent inflammatory responses to an aluminum salt adjuvant may influence vaccine efficacy during infancy and that environment factors or other early-life exposures (through stimulation of various TLR and NOD-like receptors) have the potential to modify subsequent immune responses, at least as they relate to cytokine production.[6]

The plasticity of neonatal immunity is also demonstrated in the context of the BCG vaccine. Early-life vaccination with BCG offers some protection against tuberculosis, but actually reduces neonatal mortality from non-BCG pathogens by 25−40%.[7] Investigators trying to elucidate the mechanism of these ancillary benefits administered BCG to 467 low birth-weight infants in Guinea-Bissau.[8] Whole blood cytokine levels were measured 4 weeks after BCG vaccination, which took place either at the time of birth or at 6 weeks of life (the local standard of care). Overall, BCG significantly increased in vitro cytokine expression (IL-1β, TNF, IFN-γ) after stimulation with purified protein derivative and other antigens. Importantly, these monocyte-derived pro-inflammatory cytokines tend to improve the T_h1 response, which is normally reduced in otherwise healthy infants.

Immune Interference From Maternal Antibodies

Beginning at the end of the second trimester of pregnancy, maternal antibody is actively transported across the placenta and protects infants during their first months of life.[9] Most maternal antibodies are of the IgG isotype and are metabolized over time. However, even low, non-neutralizing titers of maternal antibodies still inhibit infant immune responses to live-attenuated, inactivated and recombinant subunit vaccines.[10] The influence of maternal antibodies on infant immunity has been best studied in the context of the measles vaccine. During the first year of life, children are protected from measles by transplacentally acquired neutralizing antibodies. In clinical studies, immunization in the presence of maternal antibodies still results in reduced mortality[11] and morbidity[12]; however, protective B cell responses fail to develop. It is hypothized that the infant B cell receptor is cross-linked to an Fc receptor which results in a negative signal that inhibits both B cell proliferation and antibody secretion.[13]

One way to overcome maternal immune interference is to administer a higher titer measles vaccine.[14,15] The results have been mixed, as the higher titer vaccine improves antibody responses but also increases mortality in female recipients.[16,17] A separate approach toward countering maternal immune interference is to administer vaccine to infants at a time when maternal antibody titers start to wane. Gans et al. evaluated neutralizing antibody responses to measles vaccine in 6-, 9-, and 12-month-old infants. Antibody responses were diminished in 6-month-old infants largely because of age-dependent maturation of immune responsiveness rather than maternal antibody interference. Neutralizing antibody titers were even lower among 9-month-old infants. However, a second dose of measles vaccine at 12–15 months boosted antibody titers in both age groups to much higher levels than those in infants receiving vaccine at only 12 months of age. In addition, T cell responses were not inhibited by maternal antibody. Thus, young infants may still benefit from immunologic synergy between maternal antibodies and their own sensitized T cells.[18]

Immature B and T Cell Function

The primary goals of vaccination are to induce antigen-specific B lymphocyte and CD8 + cytotoxic T lymphocyte responses. Functional antibody responses mediated by B cells have the capacity to prevent or reduce the burden of infection by binding to the organism and triggering opsonophagocytosis or neutralizing virulence factors. Antigen-specific cytotoxic T cell responses directly or indirectly kill infected cells, thereby limiting the organism's ability to spread. Unfortunately, these responses are not as mature or robust in the neonate or young infant.[19]

The human antibody repertoire is enhanced by variable gene segment usage, high junctional diversity, and somatic hypermutation. Molecular restrictions during fetal life limit this junctional diversity. In a study of RSV-infected infants, Williams et al.[20] analyzed the molecular determinants of B cell responses. RSV-specific antibody responses in infants less than 3 months old exhibited a biased antibody repertoire that was distinct from adult responses, while infants older than 3 months had an antibody repertoire more similar to that of adults. Mutational analysis revealed that the younger infants harbored fewer somatic hypermutations in both framework and complementarity-determining regions of their antibodies than adults. This lack of somatic hypermutation in response to antigen stimulation likely contributes to the more limited repertoire of functional antibody responses seen in very young infants. Still, there may be some benefit to this limited diversity, as neonatal B cell responses appear to be aimed at generating memory responses at the expense of plasma-cell responses.[19] Therefore, the lack of somatic hypermutation may provide the basis for preferential neonatal differentiation towards memory responses.[21–23]

The immune response of the young infant is also constrained by the relative abundance of immature/transitional B and T cells. Recent thymic emigrants (RTEs) (T lymphocytes that have recently been released by the thymus) represent a large proportion of T cells in the infant circulation.[24] These RTEs proliferate less and produce less IL-2 and IFN-γ than other T-lymphocytes. They are, as a result, functionally immature. Similarly, transitional B cells that have been recently released from the bone marrow are also found in abundance in the young infant's circulation. These B cells are similarly limited in function, making the infant more vulnerable to infection.[25]

The limitations of infant immunity should dictate the design of vaccines aimed at preventing neonatal and early infant disease. One example of how knowledge of neonatal immunity has guided vaccine development comes in the context of infants at high-risk for *Haemophilus influenzae* type B (Hib) disease (e.g., Alaskan natives, American Indians). In these populations, the administration of a vaccine that conjugates the Hib polysaccharide to the outer membrane protein of meningococcus (PRP-OMP) induces a quicker immune response than other conjugates because it activates dendritic cells through stimulation of TLR2.[26,27] However, this elicits a lower overall antibody response than other Hib conjugates (i.e., CRM, tetanus), as the memory B cell pool responses are reduced and less readily boosted. Thus, additional doses with CRM or tetanus Hib conjugates are recommended to complete the primary series.

Vaccine development for young infants is challenging on account of the fundamental differences from older children and adults in innate and adaptive immunity, as well as the complicating factor of immune interference by maternally derived antibodies. While these challenges are transient, the period of risk for many infectious diseases coincides with that of diminished or altered immune responsiveness. Thus, to better optimize the infant immunization schedule, studies are needed to: (1) define better antigen delivery routes (e.g., mucosal, subcutaneous, intramuscular); (2) characterize the impact and safety of new adjuvant systems (e.g., novel oil-in-water emulsions, TLR-specific agonists); and (3) identify with greater precision the time at which maternal antibodies no longer interfere with vaccine responsiveness.

PREGNANT WOMEN

Pregnant women comprise a target population for vaccines that presents unique challenges but also great potential for protection not only of the mother herself but her infant as well.[28] In this section we discuss the complexities of determining the burden of vaccine preventable diseases in mothers and infants, maternal vaccine responses, the efficiency of transplacental antibody transport and its impact on infant immune responses, vaccine efficacy and safety in both pregnant women and their infants, and areas where additional research is needed. We will primarily use influenza vaccines as a basis for discussion, as it is the most extensively studied in this population.

Disease Burden

Influenza, malaria, hepatitis E, listeria, and herpes simplex infections can be particularly severe during pregnancy.[29] Dramatic anatomic and physiologic changes in addition to hormonal and immunologic fluctuations that occur during pregnancy can impact disease burden. A pregnant women at 38−42 weeks gestation who is infected with influenza has nearly five times the odds of having an adverse cardiopulmonary event compared with women in the postpartum period.[30] Data from the Canadian Institute of Health Information has also shown that healthy pregnant women in Canada have elevated influenza-related hospitalization rates equal to those in 65- to 69-year-old individuals.[31] The most comprehensive data on influenza burden among pregnant women were obtained during the H1N1 pandemic of 2009. During the pandemic, pregnant women were at significantly increased risk for hospitalization, intensive care unit admission and death.[32] While pregnant women only accounted for 1% of the US population in 2009, they accounted for 5% of H1N1 related deaths.[33] It is thought this increased susceptibility to severe disease is partly due to a diminished respiratory reserve during the later stages of pregnancy. In addition, more than 30% of pregnant women have comorbidities, such as asthma, diabetes, and obesity,[34] all of which can predispose to increased influenza severity.

Data on the impact of seasonal influenza infection on pregnant women in low- and middle-income countries are scarce. There are, however, some randomized controlled studies in resource-limited settings that provide burden estimates. Zaman et al., e.g., reported that 36% of febrile respiratory illnesses in pregnant women from Bangladesh was attributable to influenza.[35] In a randomized placebo-controlled influenza vaccine study in pregnant women in Soweto, South Africa, Madhi et al. found that 3.6% of HIV-uninfected pregnant women and 17% of HIV-infected pregnant women in the placebo group had laboratory confirmed influenza during the peak influenza season. Although this study enrolled more than 2000 pregnant women, it was not of sufficient size to evaluate the frequency of hospitalization, intensive care unit admissions or death. Additional influenza vaccine trials in pregnant women are ongoing in Nepal and Mali and should provide estimates of influenza attack rates in those populations, but may be underpowered to provide a full picture of the disease burden.[36] The absence of detailed influenza burden estimates makes it difficult for policymakers to project the impact of maternal influenza immunization and determine the value of a recommendation for universal immunization of pregnant women.

As outlined earlier, infants have an immature immune system incapable of fully responding to pathogens. Maternal antibody can supplement the infant's immune system during this time of vulnerability, prior to protection afforded by routine vaccinations.[37] There are a number of examples where maternal immunization has protected in infants from infectious diseases. As early as 1846, during a measles outbreak on the Faroe Islands, it was discovered that pregnant mothers who survived measles conferred immunity to their infants. In 1879, maternal immunization with vaccinia was found to protect infants from smallpox. Then, in 1938, maternal immunization with whole cell pertussis vaccine was shown to reduce the number of infants subsequently infected with *Bordetella pertussis*.[38] In 1961, universal maternal immunization with tetanus toxoid was recommended. In the ensuing decades, routine vaccination of pregnant women against tetanus has markedly reduced the global burden of neonatal tetanus disease.[39]

Surveillance data on the burden of vaccine preventable diseases among infants living in developed countries are collected and reported by national surveillance authorities such as the Centers for Disease Control and Prevention in the United States and Public Health England in the United Kingdom and by multi-country surveillance systems such as Eurosurveillance and the World Health Organization. Still, the precise numbers of infants afflicted with vaccine preventable diseases can be difficult to determine and depends on the ability to define a population, laboratory diagnostic expertise and available financial and personnel resources. However, in the same way that maternal disease burden was estimated, infant disease burden can also be measured in the setting of clinical trials. For example, Madhi et al.[40] studied a population of more than 2000 pregnant women randomized to receive either an influenza or placebo vaccine. Of the infants born to mothers who received placebo, 3.6% were diagnosed with laboratory confirmed influenza. There were also 88 infants born to HIV-infected mothers in the placebo group, of whom 6.8% had laboratory confirmed influenza. None of the infants were hospitalized for influenza; however, the sample size was not large enough to capture the full range of influenza disease.

Active surveillance studies as well as secondary data analyses have further confirmed the notion that children less than 6 months of age have a significant burden of influenza.[41] An analysis of the Tennessee Medicaid database in the 1990s revealed that healthy children younger than 1-year old were hospitalized for influenza at rates approaching those of high-risk adults.[42] Data from resource-limited settings shows much of the same.[43] In Bangladesh, 31% of infants younger than 6 months had symptomatic, laboratory confirmed influenza virus infection.[44] In The Gambia, 16% of children younger than 3 months who were hospitalized with respiratory symptoms were infected with influenza virus.[45] In Nepal, 11% of children younger than 2 years who were seen for clinical pneumonia had laboratory evidence of influenza as confirmed by real time polymerase chain reaction (RT-PCR) testing.[46] And in Thailand, children younger than 1 year of age were found to have six times the risk of hospitalization for influenza pneumonia compared to the general population.[47]

Given the consistently high estimates across regions, even from limited samples, it may be of greater public health benefit to implement universal immunization programs and then measure the decline in incidence rates. This approach presumes that a comprehensive assessment of the disease burden prior to vaccination has already been performed. An example comes from the Gambia where routine immunization with the Hib polysaccharide-tetanus toxoid conjugate vaccine was introduced nationally in May of 1997. Vaccine efficacy was determined using a case-control method, and vaccine coverage and population denominators for incidence rates were determined by cluster sample survey. Prevalence of Hib carriage was also ascertained in a subpopulation of the study group. Between May of 1997 and April of 2002, a total of 5984 children were evaluated for Hib infection. Forty-nine children had Hib disease, 36 of whom had meningitis. Five years after the Hib vaccine was introduced, annual incidence of Hib meningitis had fallen from more than 200 per 100,000 children less than 1-year old to 0 per 100,000. The prevalence of Hib carriage also decreased from 12% to 0.25%.[48] The same strategy was adopted in Indonesia and Bangladesh with similar results.[49]

Maternal Antibody Transfer

There are a number of maternal factors that impact placental antibody transfer to the fetus, particularly in the context of maternal immunization. For example, it has been conclusively shown that co-infections like HIV and malaria in pregnant women either impair or competitively bind Fc receptors and thereby reduce the efficiency of placental antibody transfer.[50,51] IgG antibody transfer also varies by subtype. IgG1, induced by protein antigens such as tetanus toxoid, are more efficiently transferred than IgG2, which is generally induced by polysaccharide antigens.[52–54] IgG transfer begins as early as 13 weeks of gestation and increases thereafter, with the largest amount transferred in the third trimester.[55] Fetal IgG concentration at term usually exceeds that in the maternal circulation.[56] However, lower birth weight infants have impaired placental IgG transfer.[57]

Maternal vaccination not only induces IgG antibodies that are transported across the placenta, but also elicits IgA, IgM, IgD antibodies that are secreted into the colostrum and milk. Upon breastfeeding, these antibodies ingested by the neonate bind and neutralize both commensal and pathogenic microbes and their virulence factors. In addition, maternal IgA facilitates antigen sampling in the neonatal intestinal mucosa by traversing M cells and delivering antigens to mucosal dendritic cells. Ingested maternal IgG can also traverse epithelial cells through a mechanism similar to that seen in transplacental antibody transport.[58]

Immunogenicity, Safety, and Efficacy of Maternal Vaccines

Immune responses to influenza vaccines in pregnant women have been evaluated in a number of studies, although many have been of small sample size, limited duration, and restricted to a specific outbreak.[59–61] Most immunogenicity studies demonstrate that vaccination of pregnant women induces an immune response similar to nonpregnant healthy young women, although two studies suggest that the immune responses may be slightly diminished in pregnant women.[62,63] In one of the largest vaccine studies of pregnant women, Madhi et al. immunized 2116 HIV-uninfected and 194 HIV-infected pregnant women.[64] At 1 month post-vaccination, sero-conversion rates and the proportion of participants with hemagglutination inhibition assay titers above the generally protective threshold of 1:40 were significantly higher among influenza vaccine than placebo recipients in both cohorts. Nonpregnant controls were not included in that study and thus could not be compared. Generally, pregnant women have experienced prior influenza infection and thus require only a single vaccination, unless the influenza strain is an avian one or one that they have not seen previously. However, despite the novelty of the H1N1 pandemic, pregnant women had an adequate immune response after only a single dose of inactivated 2009 H1N1 influenza vaccine containing 25 micrograms of hemagglutinin; efficient transplacental transfer of antibody was also documented.[61]

Studies have also been designed and executed for the determination of optimal timing of influenza immunization during pregnancy to ensure maximal transfer of antibodies to the infant. In one study, vaccine immunogenicity was tested serially throughout gestation in 239 women. Seroconversion rates were lowest in the first trimester (54.8%) and immediately postpartum (54.8%) while they were highest in the late third trimester (69.6%) and late postpartum (69.4%); however, these differences were not statistically significant. Interestingly, higher baseline antibody levels and vaccination against influenza in the previous year were both significantly associated with reduced odds of seroconversion.[65]

Vaccine safety in both pregnant women and their infants is critical for the success of a vaccine. However, safety assessments first require that underlying rates of adverse events during pregnancy be established, as they are relatively common (Table 8.2). From ovum fertilization to uterine implantation, teratogens can potentially kill the conceptus or retard its growth. Between 2 and 9 weeks post-conception, defects in organogenesis can occur. Then from 9 weeks until term, the fetus grows, differentiates and matures and is less vulnerable to teratogens. The optimal time for immunization in a pregnant woman could therefore be calculated by factoring in knowledge about the natural history of gestation, seasonality of a particular infectious disease, risks of infection to mother and infant and immunogenicity of the vaccine. In the previously cited Madhi et al. study there were no significant differences in rates of miscarriage, stillbirth, premature birth, or low birth weight infants between vaccinated and placebo groups among either HIV-uninfected or HIV-infected mothers. In addition, there were no significant local or systemic adverse events reported in the influenza vaccine recipients. Additional, large safety cohort studies of the H1N1 vaccine also

TABLE 8.2 Critical Gestational Time Periods for Teratogenesis

Period	Age Weeks[a]	Teratogenic Potential
Before implantation	0–2	Kills the embryo or no effect ("All or None").
Embryonic	2–9	May affect organogenesis and cause major defects in organs.
Fetal	9-term	May affect growth, differentiation, maturation.

The critical times for the effects of teratogens on fetal development are divided into three periods.
[a]*Weeks since fertilization.*
Source: Adapted from Bednarczyk et al. *Am J Obstet Gynecol* 2012;207(3 Suppl.):S38–46.

demonstrated an excellent safety profile among pregnant women.[66,67] In the Madhi et al. trial, vaccine efficacy for prevention of laboratory confirmed influenza was approximately 57% in both HIV-uninfected and HIV-infected mothers. Efficacy for the prevention of laboratory-confirmed influenza in infants up to 6 months old was 48% and 27% in those born to mothers with and without HIV infection, respectively. In general, influenza vaccine was immunogenic in both HIV-uninfected and HIV-infected pregnant women and provided partial protection against confirmed influenza in both groups of women and in infants who were born to HIV-uninfected mothers.

Attitudes Toward Maternal Vaccination

Even though professional societies and governing organizations have issued recommendations for routine immunization of pregnant women with tetanus, diphtheria, acellular pertussis (Tdap) vaccine, and influenza vaccine, the practice of maternal vaccination has not been widely accepted by the general public and has not become a priority among medical professionals. Despite encouraging data from post-licensure studies that show perinatal use of influenza vaccines is both safe and efficacious, maternal influenza vaccination coverage is estimated to be only 50% in the United States.[68] However, the 2009 H1N1 pandemic changed some attitudes and behaviors among health care providers and their pregnant patients.[69] It is hoped that the momentum in improved public perception will carry forward as maternal vaccination represents one of the most promising ways in which maternal and infant health may be preserved.

THE IMMUNOCOMPROMISED

The latter half of the 20th century has witnessed considerable growth in the population of immunocompromised individuals, largely because of the increasing use of novel chemotherapeutic and immunomodulatory agents. In turn, new vaccines either are being developed or have been recently licensed for some of the most virulent pathogens that cause disease in immunocompromised patients (e.g., cytomegalovirus (CMV), varicella zoster virus (VZV)).[70–72] However, the immunocompromised population is heterogeneous and the clinical and immunologic characteristics differ greatly across various immunosuppressive conditions. Some of this diversity is a consequence of the advancement of cancer treatments from older chemo- and radiotherapies to newer monoclonal antibodies and targeted drugs like tyrosine kinase inhibitors.[73] Despite these advancements, the number of clinical trials assessing vaccine responses in patients who receive these modern therapies is small. The studies that have been performed have largely been conducted among patients with hematological malignancies.[74]

Cancer patients are at greatest risk for infections and their most serious sequelae because they are often immunosuppressed from both their disease and treatment.[75] In addition, antibody titers to vaccine-preventable diseases wane rapidly after undergoing anticancer treatment.[76,77] Although vaccines could prevent a number of infections in cancer patients, vaccine coverage is less than optimal in this population. Data from the Behavioral Risk Factor Surveillance System found that 42% of cancer survivors did not receive an influenza vaccination in 2009, and that 52% reported never receiving a pneumococcal vaccination.[78] In addition, the Surveillance, Epidemiology and End Results program database, in conjunction with Medicare data, shows that breast cancer survivors aged 65 years or older are less likely to receive an influenza vaccination than noncancer controls of similar age.[79]

Recommended Vaccines

The Infectious Disease Society of America offers guidelines—according to strength of recommendation and supporting evidence—for vaccination in the immunocompromised.[74] Live attenuated vaccines (e.g., VZV, rotavirus, measles, mumps, rubella) are contraindicated in actively immunosuppressed patients because of an increased risk of developing the disease and/or prolonged shedding of the vaccine virus.[80] It is therefore recommended that patients be vaccinated prior to immunosuppression, if at all feasible, and that live vaccines be administered more than 4 weeks before immunosuppression but be avoided entirely within 2 weeks of initiating immunosuppression. The guidelines also recommend that immunocompetent individuals sharing a household with immunocompromised patients generally receive inactivated vaccines. However, there are some exceptions when those healthy immunocompetent individuals should receive live vaccines according to the CDC schedule.

Before proceeding with administration of any vaccine, a recent medication list and allergy history should be elicited from the patient. Some recommend that baseline white blood cell counts also be in the normal range or at least within reasonable limits. All agree that vaccine recipients should not have an active infection or be receiving immunosuppressive drugs or chemotherapy at the time of vaccination.[75] After these contraindications have been considered, several inactivated, subunit or virus like particle vaccines can be safely administered according to the usual doses and schedules. These vaccines include the inactivated or recombinant influenza vaccine, the 13- or 23-valent pneumococcal vaccine, the Tdap vaccine and the HPV vaccines in individuals less than 26 years old.[75] These vaccines can be safety administered to immuncompromised subjects but they may not be particularly immunogenic. Given their low risk profile, these vaccines should still be administered to all cancer and transplant patients who have completed therapy at least 3 months before vaccination. In general, the usual vaccine doses and schedules are recommended.[74,75] In those who receive treatment with anti-B cell antibodies, vaccination should be delayed for at least 6 months after the last dose to allow for reconstitution of the B cell population.

Several vaccines are being developed for a variety of populations but are of particular relevance to immunocompromised individuals. High-dose influenza vaccines have been licensed for use in those older than 65 years, as they have been shown to be more immunogenic and effective in older adults living in both community settings and long-term care facilities.[81,82] However, they also have demonstrated improved immunogenicity compared to standard vaccines in immunosuppressed children.[83,84] Transplant recipients will need vaccines that prevent the reactivation of latent viruses and protect against severe disease particularly as they often have suppressed cellular immunity. One of those latent viruses is CMV for which vaccines are also being developed.[85] A recent study has also shown that an adjuvanted VZV glycoprotein E subunit vaccine was 97% efficacious over 3 years of follow up in a cohort of older adults.[72] As the vaccine also has an excellent safety profile and is inactivated, it should be safe for use in immunocompromised individuals, although the studies in this population have yet to be done. With the advent of modern biologics and the success of hematopoietic and solid organ transplatation, vaccination of immunocompromised hosts will become a larger aspect of public health. It will be increasingly important to understand the precise mechanisms of immunosuppression, the timeline of immunologic recovery, and the roles of adjuvants and antigen dosing and delivery to better protect people who are most vulnerable to severe infections.

OLDER ADULTS

The population of older adults is rapidly growing. By 2050, the US population aged 65 years and over is projected to be 83.7 million, almost double the estimated population of 43.1 million in 2012. Similar increases are projected in the global population with people over 60 years rising from 11% to 22% of the world population by 2050.[86] This increase will be accompanied by a rise in age-related diseases including infections, cancer, cardiovascular and neuro-degenerative diseases. Some of the increased risk for these diseases is partially due to immunosenescence: an age-associated decline in the function of the immune system. Immunosenescence affects both innate and adaptive immunity and impairs host responses to both pathogens and vaccines.[86] Much of the effects can be seen on T cell populations as this can lead to an inverse CD4/CD8 T cell ratio, relative loss in the number of naïve T cells (due to thymic involution), rise in terminally differentiated T cells, oligoclonal expansion of virus-specific T cells but overall restricted diversity of T cells. B cell immunity can also suffer, as defects in isotype switching and somatic hypermutation are more common in older adults.[87] A study that assessed the levels of vaccine-specific plasmablasts 1 week after trivalent influenza vaccination (TIV) in younger (18−51 years) and older adults (older than 70 years) found a reduction in the number of plasmablasts in older adults, but a similar ratio of secreted IgG per plasmablast and avidity of plasmablast-derived antibodies across the two age groups.[88] As the challenges to inducing protective immune responses in older adults are formidable, new vaccine strategies will need to be devised for this special population.

Since US public health officials first recommended annual influenza vaccination for all adults over the age of 65, older adults have been considered a special population.[89] These recommendations were largely based on the premise that influenza vaccines were effective in preventing clinical illness in younger subjects and would, by extrapolation, reduce the risk of death among the aged and chronically ill.[90] However, vaccine efficacy trials had not yet been conducted in older adults. Subsequent observational studies have proven that assessment of the impact of influenza vaccination on all-cause hospitalizations and deaths in older adults is particularly challenging. Early influenza vaccine efficacy studies were performed in military populations of young and healthy males, but it was unclear how these results could be extrapolated to older populations. Traditionally, nasopharyngeal swab culture was used as the gold-standard for influenza diagnosis. However, older adults tended to have lower viral titers in their respiratory secretions than younger adults and children.[91] In a study of older adults with serologically confirmed influenza, culture only identified half of the infections.[92] When compared to PCR as the gold standard, the sensitivity of culture fell even lower to 21−50%.[93]

Three randomized clinical trials have evaluated the efficacy of TIVs in older adults. Two of the studies used both influenza-like illness and serologic conversion as endpoints.[94−96] Other than these trials, case-control and cohort studies have been the main way to evaluate influenza vaccine effectiveness in older adults. A recent Cochrane review of 75 studies found that influenza vaccines afford only modest protection in older adults in the community setting.[97] One of the limitations in interpreting these findings, particularly among clinical trials, is the tendency to use multiple outcomes.[95] For example, in a clinical trial evaluating the efficacy of influenza vaccine in healthy adults, three distinct end-points were used: serologically confirmed influenza, febrile respiratory tract illness, and upper respiratory infection. Vaccine efficacy varied widely by end-point: 86% for laboratory-confirmed influenza, 34% for febrile respiratory illnesses, and only 10% for upper respiratory infection.[98]

We and others have used hospital discharge codes to assess the impact of influenza vaccine on the number of excess cases of pneumonia, influenza or respiratory admissions in older populations. This method allows the assessment of much larger databases to increase the sample size of the population studied, although it limits the ability to determine whether individual patients have laboratory-confirmed influenza. For example, in one of our studies we found that only 28.2% of the hospitalized individuals older than 50 years who had RT-PCR confirmed influenza were given pneumonia or influenza discharge codes, while another 69.2% were given other codes for respiratory and circulatory disorders. Those who were RT-PCR negative were given similar discharge codes, with 28.3% receiving pneumonia and influenza codes and 67.2% given other respiratory and circulatory diagnostic codes.[99] Thus, it is not possible to determine, by discharge codes alone, which patients had laboratory confirmed influenza and which ones did not, generating misclassification bias and possibly overestimating vaccine effectiveness. In other words, if an influenza vaccine were 50% effective at preventing all cardiopulmonary hospitalizations, it would have to prevent diseases not caused by influenza, which is highly unlikely to occur.

Vaccine Uptake

The uptake of influenza vaccines varies greatly by socioeconomic status, race and level of frailty. Frailty, a multi-factorial syndrome that represents a reduction in physiological reserve and an inability to resist stressors, is increasingly been assessed as a marker for susceptibility to influenza disease and for vaccine responses.[100–102] In addition, frailty has been shown to predict vaccine response to the polysaccharide pneumococcal vaccines better than age[103] and is a confounder in influenza vaccine efficacy studies.[104,105]

One of the biggest challenges to accurately monitoring vaccine uptake in older populations is that vaccines are being administered by nontraditional providers with increasing frequency. In the past, most patients received vaccines either from their primary care provider or at public health clinics. Now, there are many places where people can be vaccinated, including pharmacies, grocery stores, employers, and large retail stores. Although expanded venues for vaccination enhance immunization rates, vaccinations delivered outside of the traditional clinical setting are often not captured by administrative databases, making assessments of uptake and effectiveness more difficult.[106] A survey by the CDC in 2011 demonstrated that nearly one quarter of adults older than 65 years were vaccinated at a nontraditional site.[107]

Based on this figure, a study that analyzes vaccine registries or insurance billing data might misclassify as many as 25% of vaccinated individuals as unvaccinated. With these concerns in mind, we sought to determine the effectiveness of TIV in older adults with confirmation of receipt at non-traditional locations. Adults older than 50 years who were hospitalized with respiratory symptoms or nonlocalizing fever were prospectively tested for influenza using RT-PCR. Those individuals who were PCR positive were classified as cases and compared to PCR negative controls. Since both groups were hospitalized, it would be expected that the cases and controls would be similar in their health care seeking behaviors. Vaccine receipt was verified with medical providers, employers, retail pharmacies, and retail groceries. The estimated overall vaccine efficacy over 2 years was 61.2%,[99] which may represent a more accurate estimate given that it includes a wider catchment of vaccinees.

New Vaccines

In an effort to overcome the effects of an aging immune system, several new vaccine approaches are being developed, such as the addition of potent new adjuvants and the administration of higher doses of vaccine. Based on several efficacy studies, a new high-dose influenza vaccine has recently been licensed in the United States, containing four times the usual amount of HA protein for each of the three influenza vaccine strains (60 micrograms of HA).[81,108,109] Although local reactions have been somewhat more frequent with the high dose, they have been of mild to moderate in intensity. In addition, oil-in-water emulsion-based adjuvants like MF59 and AS03 have been shown to improve the immunogenicity of a number of vaccines in individuals of different ages. An influenza vaccine containing MF-59 has been licensed in Europe and has been shown to be safe after being used by more than 45 million people.[110] A recent review of 64 clinical trials of the MF59-adjuvanted influenza vaccine found it to be safe after being used in almost 27,000 individuals ranging in age from 6 months to 100 years. Solicited local and systemic reactions up to 3 days after first vaccination were higher in individuals who received adjuvanted vaccine, though they were mild and transient.[111] Routine vaccination against influenza has been recommended for years and older adults would likely benefit from newer, more immunogenic vaccines. Until these new vaccines become available, however, currently available vaccines like TIV should be administered to those of advanced age to reduce their excess morbidity and mortality from vaccine preventable diseases.

REGULATORY CONSIDERATIONS

All vaccines in the United States are developed under the oversight of the Food and Drug Administration Center for Biologics Evaluation and Research

(CBER). In its role as a licensing authority, CBER provides guidance to industry on the development, testing, and post-marketing safety reporting of human drug and biologic products, including vaccines. These documents expand on the requirements set forth in the Code of Federal Regulations (specifically, 21 CFR) to provide guidance on the data needed to support vaccine licensure, labeling and assessment of impact on special populations. Similarly, in the European Union, the European Medicines Agency Committee for Medicinal Products for Human Use provides oversight for the clinical evaluation of new vaccines. Guidance is provided on characterization of the immunogenicity, durability, dosing, schedule, and the need for booster doses.[112] Importantly, demonstration of protective efficacy is not necessary for all vaccines. However, the use correlates of protection for licensure is generally contingent on binding commitments to conduct post-licensure studies of vaccine effectiveness. For vaccines that may be co-administered with other already licensed vaccines, the assessment of immune interference must be considered. In addition, extensive general safety data must be provided that provides guidance on rates of anticipated adverse events and frequency of serious complications following vaccination.

Since the target population for many vaccines in development includes women of childbearing potential, the evaluation of a vaccine's developmental toxicity profile is warranted. Therefore, in 2006, CBER issued guidance for preclinical studies that aids in the application of 21 CFR and the ICH S5A Guidance for the Detection of Toxicity to Reproduction. This guidance document focused on vaccines intended for adolescent and adult populations, rather than infancy and childhood, given the potential for immunization of pregnant women. For products that are specifically intended for maternal immunization or use in women of childbearing potential, it is recommended that preclinical developmental toxicity data be available prior to the initiation of any clinical trial that enrolls these populations. However, if these data are not available, women may be screened for pregnancy and instructed to use contraception during the clinical trial. Preclinical developmental toxicity has to be performed as well and meet the following requirements: demonstration of an immune response in the pregnant female animal, verification of fetal exposure to maternal antibodies and evaluation of toxic effects of not only the antigen but also the adjuvant, additives, and residuals present in the final formulation of the vaccine. It is also recommended that one or several doses of vaccine be given during organogenesis. This approach also provides high-level antibody exposure to the fetus for the duration of gestation.

CONCLUSION

Taken together, it is clear that special populations such as young infants, pregnant women, immunocompromised persons and older adults require special considerations when designing, developing, and delivering vaccines. The process to vaccine licensure should take into account the unique demography and immunologic milieu of each population. It is also clear that the same rigor used for the regulatory approval of medicinal agents should be used for vaccines. Given the recent increase in the number of licensed vaccines either recommended or available for use in special populations, preclinical toxicity and clinical safety data will be critical as new vaccines enter the market. However, as tailored vaccines are developed, there should be no hesitation in administering vaccines to all populations according to current recommendations, as what makes these populations special is their particular vulnerability to infectious diseases.

REFERENCES

1. Lucas WP, Amoss HL. Vaccine treatment in the prevention of dysentery in infants. *J Exp Med* 1911;**13**(5):486−94.
2. Luca S, Mihaescu T. History of BCG vaccine. *Maedica (Buchar)* 2013;**8**(1):53−8.
3. Calmette A, et al. *La vaccination preventive contre la tuberculose par le "BCG,"* 250. Paris: Masson et cie; 1927. p. 11.
4. Kollmann TR, et al. Innate immune function by toll-like receptors: distinct responses in newborns and the elderly. *Immunity* 2012;**37**(5):771−83.
5. Shey MS, et al. Maturation of innate responses to mycobacteria over the first nine months of life. *J Immunol* 2014;**192**(10):4833−43.
6. Lisciandro JG, et al. Ontogeny of toll-like and NOD-like receptor-mediated innate immune responses in Papua New Guinean infants. *PLoS One* 2012;**7**(5):e36793.
7. Shann F. The non-specific effects of vaccines. *Arch Dis Child* 2010;**95**(9):662−7.
8. Jensen KJ, et al. Heterologous immunological effects of early BCG vaccination in low-birth-weight infants in Guinea-Bissau: a randomized-controlled trial. *J Infect Dis* 2015;**211**(6):956−67.
9. Kohler PF, Farr RS. Elevation of cord over maternal IgG immunoglobulin: evidence for an active placental IgG transport. *Nature* 1966;**210**(5040):1070−1.
10. Niewiesk S. Maternal antibodies: clinical significance, mechanism of interference with immune responses, and possible vaccination strategies. *Front Immunol* 2014;**5**:446.
11. Samb B, et al. Serologic status and measles attack rates among vaccinated and unvaccinated children in rural Senegal. *Pediatr Infect Dis J* 1995;**14**(3):203−9.
12. Gans H, et al. Immune responses to measles and mumps vaccination of infants at 6, 9, and 12 months. *J Infect Dis* 2001;**184**(7):817−26.
13. Kim D, Niewiesk S. Sidestepping maternal antibody: a lesson from measles virus vaccination. *Expert Rev Clin Immunol* 2011;**7**(5):557−9.
14. Whittle H, et al. Trial of high-dose Edmonston-Zagreb measles vaccine in The Gambia: antibody response and side-effects. *Lancet* 1988;**2**(8615):811−14.
15. Whittle HC, et al. Effects of dose and strain of vaccine on success of measles vaccination of infants aged 4−5 months. *Lancet* 1988;**1**(8592):963−6.
16. Seng R, et al. Increased long term mortality associated with rash after early measles vaccination in rural Senegal. *Pediatr Infect Dis J* 1999;**18**(1):48−52.
17. Garenne M, et al. Child mortality after high-titre measles vaccines: prospective study in Senegal. *Lancet* 1991;**338**(8772):903−7.

18. Gans H, et al. Measles and mumps vaccination as a model to investigate the developing immune system: passive and active immunity during the first year of life. *Vaccine* 2003;**21** (24):3398−405.

19. Prabhu Das M, et al. Challenges in infant immunity: implications for responses to infection and vaccines. *Nat Immunol* 2011;**12**(3):189−94.

20. Williams JV, et al. The human neonatal B cell response to respiratory syncytial virus uses a biased antibody variable gene repertoire that lacks somatic mutations. *Mol Immunol* 2009;**47**(2−3):407−14.

21. Smith KG, et al. The extent of affinity maturation differs between the memory and antibody-forming cell compartments in the primary immune response. *EMBO J* 1997;**16** (11):2996−3006.

22. Bryant VL, et al. Cytokine-mediated regulation of human B cell differentiation into Ig-secreting cells: predominant role of IL-21 produced by CXCR5 + T follicular helper cells. *J Immunol* 2007;**179**(12):8180−90.

23. Gatto D, et al. Complement receptors regulate differentiation of bone marrow plasma cell precursors expressing transcription factors Blimp-1 and XBP-1. *J Exp Med* 2005;**201** (6):993−1005.

24. Haines CJ, et al. Human CD4 + T cell recent thymic emigrants are identified by protein tyrosine kinase 7 and have reduced immune function. *J Exp Med* 2009;**206**(2):275−85.

25. Basha S, Surendran N, Pichichero M. Immune responses in neonates. *Expert Rev Clin Immunol* 2014;**10**(9):1171−84.

26. Latz E, et al. *Haemophilus influenzae* type B-outer membrane protein complex glycoconju-gate vaccine induces cytokine production by engaging human toll-like receptor 2 (TLR2) and requires the presence of TLR2 for optimal immunogenicity. *J Immunol* 2004;**172** (4):2431−8.

27. Decker MD, et al. Comparative trial in infants of four conjugate *Haemophilus influenzae* type B vaccines. *J Pediatr* 1992;**120**(2 Pt 1):184−9.

28. Lindsey B, Kampmann B, Jones C. Maternal immunization as a strategy to decrease susceptibility to infection in newborn infants. *Curr Opin Infect Dis* 2013;**26**(3):248−53.

29. Kourtis AP, Read JS, Jamieson DJ. Pregnancy and infection. *N Engl J Med* 2014;**371** (11):1077.

30. Neuzil KM, et al. Impact of influenza on acute cardiopulmonary hospitalizations in pregnant women. *Am J Epidemiol* 1998;**148**(11):1094−102.

31. Schanzer DL, Langley JM, Tam TW. Influenza-attributed hospitalization rates among pregnant women in Canada 1994−2000. *J Obstet Gynaecol Can* 2007;**29**(8):622−9.

32. Mosby LG, Rasmussen SA, Jamieson DJ. 2009 pandemic influenza A (H1N1) in pregnancy: a systematic review of the literature. *Am J Obstet Gynecol* 2011;**205**(1):10−18.

33. Siston AM, et al. Pandemic 2009 influenza A (H1N1) virus illness among pregnant women in the United States. *JAMA* 2010;**303**(15):1517−25.

34. Mosby LG, et al. The Centers for Disease Control and Prevention's maternal health response to 2009 H1N1 influenza. *Am J Obstet Gynecol* 2011;**204**(6 Suppl. 1):S7−12.

35. Chan GJ, et al. The effect of intrapartum antibiotics on early-onset neonatal sepsis in Dhaka, Bangladesh: a propensity score matched analysis. *BMC Pediatr* 2014;**14**:104.

36. Omer SB, et al. Three randomized trials of maternal influenza immunization in Mali, Nepal, and South Africa: methods and expectations. *Vaccine* 2015;**33**(32):3801−12.

37. Englund JA. The influence of maternal immunization on infant immune responses. *J Comp Pathol* 2007;**137**(Suppl. 1):S16−19.

38. Lichty JA, Slavin B, Bradford WL. An attempt to increase resistance to pertussis in newborn infants by immunizing their mothers during pregnancy. *J Clin Invest* 1938;**17**(5):613–21.

39. Healy CM. Vaccines in pregnant women and research initiatives. *Clin Obstet Gynecol* 2012;**55**(2):474–86.

40. Madhi SA, Nunes MC, Cutland CL. Influenza vaccination of pregnant women and protection of their infants. *N Engl J Med* 2014;**371**(24):2340.

41. Poehling KA, et al. The underrecognized burden of influenza in young children. *N Engl J Med* 2006;**355**(1):31–40.

42. Neuzil KM, et al. The effect of influenza on hospitalizations, outpatient visits, and courses of antibiotics in children. *N Engl J Med* 2000;**342**(4):225–31.

43. Ortiz JR, Englund JA, Neuzil KM. Influenza vaccine for pregnant women in resource-constrained countries: a review of the evidence to inform policy decisions. *Vaccine* 2011;**29**(27):4439–52.

44. Henkle E, et al. The effect of exclusive breast-feeding on respiratory illness in young infants in a maternal immunization trial in Bangladesh. *Pediatr Infect Dis J* 2013;**32**(5):431–5.

45. Mulholland EK, et al. Etiology of serious infections in young Gambian infants. *Pediatr Infect Dis J* 1999;**18**(10 Suppl.):S35–41.

46. Mathisen M, et al. RNA viruses in community-acquired childhood pneumonia in semi-urban Nepal: a cross-sectional study. *BMC Med* 2009;**7**:35.

47. Simmerman JM, et al. The cost of influenza in Thailand. *Vaccine* 2006;**24**(20):4417–26.

48. Mulholland EK, Adegbola RA. The Gambian *Haemophilus influenzae* type B vaccine trial: what does it tell us about the burden of *Haemophilus influenzae* type B disease? *Pediatr Infect Dis J* 1998;**17**(9 Suppl.):S123–5.

49. Mulholland EK. Use of vaccine trials to estimate burden of disease. *J Health Popul Nutr* 2004;**22**(3):257–67.

50. de Moraes-Pinto MI, et al. Placental antibody transfer: influence of maternal HIV infection and placental malaria. *Arch Dis Child Fetal Neonatal Ed* 1998;**79**(3):F202–5.

51. Hartter HK, et al. Placental transfer and decay of maternally acquired antimeasles antibodies in Nigerian children. *Pediatr Infect Dis J* 2000;**19**(7):635–41.

52. Glezen WP, Alpers M. Maternal immunization. *Clin Infect Dis* 1999;**28**(2):219–24.

53. Costa-Carvalho BT, et al. Transfer of IgG subclasses across placenta in term and preterm newborns. *Braz J Med Biol Res* 1996;**29**(2):201–4.

54. van den Berg JP, et al. Transplacental transport of IgG antibodies specific for pertussis, diphtheria, tetanus, *Haemophilus influenzae* type B, and *Neisseria meningitidis* serogroup C is lower in preterm compared with term infants. *Pediatr Infect Dis J* 2010;**29**(9):801–5.

55. Saji F, et al. Dynamics of immunoglobulins at the feto-maternal interface. *Rev Reprod* 1999;**4**(2):81–9.

56. Linder N, Ohel G. In utero vaccination. *Clin Perinatol* 1994;**21**(3):663–74.

57. Wesumperuma HL, et al. The influence of prematurity and low birthweight on transplacental antibody transfer in Sri Lanka. *Ann Trop Med Parasitol* 1999;**93**(2):169–77.

58. Faucette AN, et al. Maternal vaccination: moving the science forward. *Hum Reprod Update* 2015;**21**(1):119–35.

59. Fisher BM, et al. Pandemic influenza A H1N1 2009 infection versus vaccination: a cohort study comparing immune responses in pregnancy. *PLoS One* 2012;**7**(3):e33048.

60. Tsatsaris V, et al. Maternal immune response and neonatal seroprotection from a single dose of a monovalent nonadjuvanted 2009 influenza A (H1N1) vaccine: a single-group trial. *Ann Intern Med* 2011;**155**(11):733−41.

61. Jackson LA, et al. Immunogenicity of an inactivated monovalent 2009 H1N1 influenza vaccine in pregnant women. *J Infect Dis* 2011;**204**(6):854−63.

62. Schlaudecker EP, et al. Pregnancy modifies the antibody response to trivalent influenza immunization. *J Infect Dis* 2012;**206**(11):1670−3.

63. Bischoff AL, et al. Altered response to A(H1N1)pnd09 vaccination in pregnant women: a single blinded randomized controlled trial. *PLoS One* 2013;**8**(4):e56700.

64. Madhi SA, et al. Influenza vaccination of pregnant women and protection of their infants. *N Engl J Med* 2014;**371**(10):918−31.

65. Sperling RS, et al. Immunogenicity of trivalent inactivated influenza vaccination received during pregnancy or postpartum. *Obstet Gynecol* 2012;**119**(3):631−9.

66. Heikkinen T, et al. Safety of MF59-adjuvanted A/H1N1 influenza vaccine in pregnancy: a comparative cohort study. *Am J Obstet Gynecol* 2012;**207**(3):177.e1−8.

67. Ludvigsson JF, et al. Influenza H1N1 vaccination and adverse pregnancy outcome. *Eur J Epidemiol* 2013;**28**(7):579−88.

68. Johnson NB, et al. CDC National Health Report: leading causes of morbidity and mortality and associated behavioral risk and protective factors − United States, 2005−2013. *MMWR Surveill Summ* 2014;**63**(Suppl. 4):3−27.

69. Halperin BA, et al. Maintaining the momentum: key factors influencing acceptance of influenza vaccination among pregnant women following the H1N1 pandemic. *Hum Vaccin Immunother* 2014;**10**(12):3629−41.

70. Kharfan-Dabaja MA, et al. A novel therapeutic cytomegalovirus DNA vaccine in allogeneic haemopoietic stem-cell transplantation: a randomised, double-blind, placebo-controlled, phase 2 trial. *Lancet Infect Dis* 2012;**12**(4):290−9.

71. Griffiths PD, et al. Cytomegalovirus glycoprotein-B vaccine with MF59 adjuvant in transplant recipients: a phase 2 randomised placebo-controlled trial. *Lancet* 2011;**377** (9773):1256−63.

72. Lal H, et al. Efficacy of an adjuvanted herpes zoster subunit vaccine in older adults. *N Engl J Med* 2015;**372**(22):2087−96.

73. Plotkin SA, Orenstein WA, Offit PA. *Vaccines.* 6th ed. Philadelphia, PA: Elsevier Saunders; 2013. xix, 1550 p.

74. Rubin LG, et al. 2013 IDSA clinical practice guideline for vaccination of the immunocompromised host. *Clin Infect Dis* 2014;**58**(3):e44−100.

75. Denlinger CS, et al. Survivorship: immunizations and prevention of infections, version 2.2014. *J Natl Compr Canc Netw* 2014;**12**(8):1098−111.

76. Kwon HJ, et al. Assessment of serologic immunity to diphtheria-tetanus-pertussis after treatment of Korean pediatric hematology and oncology patients. *J Korean Med Sci* 2012;**27**(1):78−83.

77. Ljungman P, et al. Vaccination of hematopoietic cell transplant recipients. *Bone Marrow Transplant* 2009;**44**(8):521−6.

78. Underwood JM, et al. Surveillance of demographic characteristics and health behaviors among adult cancer survivors − Behavioral Risk Factor Surveillance System, United States, 2009. *MMWR Surveill Summ* 2012;**61**(1):1−23.

79. Snyder CF, et al. Comparing care for breast cancer survivors to non-cancer controls: a five-year longitudinal study. *J Gen Intern Med* 2009;**24**(4):469−74.

80. Rubin LG, et al. 2013 IDSA clinical practice guideline for vaccination of the immuno-compromised host. *Clin Infect Dis* 2014;**58**(3):309–18.

81. Nace DA, et al. Randomized, controlled trial of high-dose influenza vaccine among frail residents of long-term care facilities. *J Infect Dis* 2015;**211**(12):1915–24.

82. DiazGranados CA, et al. Efficacy of high-dose versus standard-dose influenza vaccine in older adults. *N Engl J Med* 2014;**371**(7):635–45.

83. McManus M, et al. Safety of high dose trivalent inactivated influenza vaccine in pediatric patients with acute lymphoblastic leukemia. *Pediatr Blood Cancer* 2014;**61**(5):815–20.

84. GiaQuinta S, et al. Randomized, double-blind comparison of standard-dose vs. high-dose trivalent inactivated influenza vaccine in pediatric solid organ transplant patients. *Pediatr Transplant* 2015;**19**(2):219–28.

85. Dasari V, Smith C, Khanna R. Recent advances in designing an effective vaccine to prevent cytomegalovirus-associated clinical diseases. *Expert Rev Vaccines* 2013;**12**(6):661–76.

86. Pera A, et al. Immunosenescence: implications for response to infection and vaccination in older people. *Maturitas* 2015;**82**(1):50–5.

87. Weinberger B, et al. Biology of immune responses to vaccines in elderly persons. *Clin Infect Dis* 2008;**46**(7):1078–84.

88. Sasaki S, et al. Limited efficacy of inactivated influenza vaccine in elderly individuals is associated with decreased production of vaccine-specific antibodies. *J Clin Invest* 2011;**121**(8):3109–19.

89. Talbot HK, Libster R, Edwards KM. Influenza vaccination for older adults. *Hum Vaccin Immunother* 2012;**8**(1):96–101.

90. Langmuir AD, Henderson DA, Serfling RE. The epidemiological basis for the control of influenza. *Am J Public Health Nations Health* 1964;**54**:563–71.

91. Walsh EE, Cox C, Falsey AR. Clinical features of influenza A virus infection in older hospitalized persons. *J Am Geriatr Soc* 2002;**50**(9):1498–503.

92. Flamaing J, et al. Viral lower respiratory tract infection in the elderly: a prospective in-hospital study. *Eur J Clin Microbiol Infect Dis* 2003;**22**(12):720–5.

93. Falsey AR, et al. Respiratory syncytial virus infection in elderly and high-risk adults. *N Engl J Med* 2005;**352**(17):1749–59.

94. Govaert TM, et al. Immune response to influenza vaccination of elderly people. A randomized double-blind placebo-controlled trial. *Vaccine* 1994;**12**(13):1185–9.

95. Praditsuwan R, et al. The efficacy and effectiveness of influenza vaccination among Thai elderly persons living in the community. *J Med Assoc Thai* 2005;**88**(2):256–64.

96. Allsup S, et al. Is influenza vaccination cost effective for healthy people between ages 65 and 74 years? A randomised controlled trial. *Vaccine* 2004;**23**(5):639–45.

97. Jefferson T, et al. Vaccines for preventing influenza in the elderly. *Cochrane Database Syst Rev* 2010;(2):CD004876.

98. Bridges CB, et al. Effectiveness and cost-benefit of influenza vaccination of healthy working adults: a randomized controlled trial. *JAMA* 2000;**284**(13):1655–63.

99. Talbot HK, et al. Effectiveness of seasonal vaccine in preventing confirmed influenza-associated hospitalizations in community dwelling older adults. *J Infect Dis* 2011;**203**(4):500–8.

100. Yao X, et al. Frailty is associated with impairment of vaccine-induced antibody response and increase in post-vaccination influenza infection in community-dwelling older adults. *Vaccine* 2011;**29**(31):5015–21.

101. Strandberg TE, Pitkala KH. Frailty in elderly people. *Lancet* 2007;**369**(9570):1328–9.

102. Rockwood K, et al. A global clinical measure of fitness and frailty in elderly people. *CMAJ* 2005;**173**(5):489–95.

103. Ridda I, et al. Immunological responses to pneumococcal vaccine in frail older people. *Vaccine* 2009;**27**(10):1628–36.

104. Jackson LA, et al. Functional status is a confounder of the association of influenza vaccine and risk of all cause mortality in seniors. *Int J Epidemiol* 2006;**35**(2):345–52.

105. Baxter R, Ray GT, Fireman BH. Effect of influenza vaccination on hospitalizations in persons aged 50 years and older. *Vaccine* 2010;**28**(45):7267–72.

106. Greene SK, et al. Accuracy of data on influenza vaccination status at four Vaccine Safety Datalink sites. *Am J Prev Med* 2009;**37**(6):552–5.

107. Centers for Disease Control and Prevention. Place of influenza vaccination among adults – United States, 2010–11 influenza season. *Morb Mortal Wkly Rep* 2011;**60**(23):781–5.

108. Falsey AR, et al. Randomized, double-blind controlled phase 3 trial comparing the immunogenicity of high-dose and standard-dose influenza vaccine in adults 65 years of age and older. *J Infect Dis* 2009;**200**(2):172–80.

109. DiazGranados CA, et al. High-dose trivalent influenza vaccine compared to standard dose vaccine in elderly adults: safety, immunogenicity and relative efficacy during the 2009–2010 season. *Vaccine* 2013;**31**(6):861–6.

110. Rappuoli R, et al. Public health. Rethinking influenza. *Science* 2009;**326**(5949):50.

111. Pellegrini M, et al. MF59-adjuvanted versus non-adjuvanted influenza vaccines: integrated analysis from a large safety database. *Vaccine* 2009;**27**(49):6959–65.

112. European Medicines Agency (EMA). *Guideline on clinical evaluation of new vaccines*. London: EMA; 2006.

Index